THE NO-GRAIN
Diet

THE NO-GRAIN
Diet

Conquer Carbohydrate Addiction and Stay Slim for Life

Dr. Joseph Mercola

WITH ALISON ROSE LEVY

DUTTON

DUTTON
Published by the Penguin Group (USA) Inc., 375 Hudson Street, New York, New York 10014, U.S.A.
Penguin Books Ltd, Registered Offices: 80 Strand, London WC2R 0RL, England
Penguin Books Australia Ltd, 250 Camberwell Road, Camberwell, Victoria 3124, Australia
Penguin Books Canada Ltd, 10 Alcorn Avenue, Toronto, Ontario, Canada M4V 3B2
Penguin Books (NZ) Ltd, Cnr Rosedale and Airborne Roads, Albany, Auckland 1310, New Zealand

Published by Dutton, a member of Penguin Group (USA) Inc.

First printing, May 2003
10 9 8 7 6

REGISTERED TRADEMARK—MARCA REGISTRADA

LIBRARY OF CONGRESS CATALOGING-IN-PUBLICATION DATA

Mercola, Joseph.
    The no-grain diet : conquer carbohydrate addiction and stay slim for life / by Joseph Mercola, with Alison Rose Levy.
        p. cm.
    Includes bibliographical references.
        ISBN 0-525-94733-7 (hc : alk paper)
        1. Low-carbohydrate diet. 2. Reducing diets. 3. Grain. I. Levy, Alison Rose. II. Title.
    RM237.73.M47 2003
    613.2'83—dc21

                                                                              2003001278

Printed in the United States of America
Set in Berkeley Book

CONTENTS

PART FOUR: Recipes

THE NO-GRAIN DIET

**There Are Three Phases to the Diet to Optimize
Weight Loss and Healthy Living:**

The
Start-Up →
Phase

The
Stabilize →
Phase

The
Sustain
Phase

(The first 3 days
of the diet)

(The next 50 days +)

(Lifelong)

**There Are Three Food Plans to Help You
Stay on the Diet and Enjoy Life More:**

The
Booster
Food Plan →

The
Core
Food Plan →

The
Advanced
Food Plan

(Easiest food plan
to follow because
it has the most
allowable foods—
it literally boosts
you on the diet)

(Faster results on
this slightly more
stringent food plan)

(Necessary for
those looking
for a lot of weight
loss quickly
because of
health reasons)

Use the Emotional Freedom Technique (EFT) to break free from
your cravings and emotional attachment to food.

*Now, turn the page and get ready to **lose weight**, **be healthy**,
and **love life!***

PART ONE

WHY A NO-GRAIN DIET?

CHAPTER 1

THE OBESITY EPIDEMIC

After more than three decades of consuming less fat and more carbohydrates, the average American is gaining weight at an alarming rate. We are eating sixty pounds more grain and thirty pounds more sweeteners than we did twenty-five years ago. The effects are clear: over two-thirds of Americans are overweight or obese. With excess weight the single, most important factor in the onset of cancer, heart disease, and diabetes, we now face an epidemic with health costs skyrocketing to $1.5 trillion. As medical experts desperately seek answers, I am thankful I can offer an effective and time-tested solution in *The No-Grain Diet.*

For over a decade, the *No-Grain Diet* has been the centerpiece of my medical practice, used by hundreds of thousands of patients who visit my wellness center and my website at *www.mercola.com.* While the medical debate has simmered below the surface of media attention, I've been quietly refining my dietary strategy with nearly miraculous results. And finally, both doctors and the general public are recognizing a growing body of scientific evidence that supports what I've advocated all along. Eating certain kinds of carbohydrates, not fats, causes escalating weight gain and wide-ranging health problems.

According to writer Gary Taubes, in his cover article in the July 7, 2002, *New York Times Magazine,* new research confirms that the USDA food pyramid, the low cholesterol heart disease diet, and the medical recommendations to eat less fat and more carbohydrates "are the cause of the rampaging epidemic of obesity in America."

The Culprits in Weight Gain

Fats aren't to blame for weight gain! In studying our endocrine system, new research I'll detail more fully in the next chapter finds that the real culprits are grains, starches, and sweets. These foods trigger a hormonal cycle of grain and sugar addiction, weight gain, and diabetes. That's why eliminating all grains, starches, and sugars for a limited period of time is the best way to reprogram your cells to burn fat. Erasing the signals that prompt you to eat will help you overcome cravings and addictive food urges. Combining these two approaches, the *No-Grain Diet* provides a comprehensive strategy that will help you rewire your physical and emotional hardware so you can lose weight and conquer carb cravings forever.

What's in a Grain?

In your body, grains, grain products, starches, and sugars have one thing in common: they rapidly turn to glucose, promote addictive eating habits, and trigger insulin release, all of which contribute to weight gain and other health problems.

Carbohydrates from grains and sugars produce a very different effect from the ones found in vegetables, which you'll enjoy on this diet. That's why it's very important to learn to distinguish between them.

Grain and sugar carbs = unhealthy foods. Vegetable carbs = healthy foods (in most cases).

Grains and grain products, including bread, flour, chips, and baked goods, are not the only sources of these detrimental carbohydrates. They are also found in:

- Many starchy vegetables, like potatoes and carrots, as well as their products
- Concentrated fruit products, like fruit juices or syrups
- The vast majority of sweeteners, and all foods containing them

Throughout this book, when I use the term *No-Grain*, I'm *not* only speaking about grains. Instead, I'll use the terms *No-Grain* and *grains* inclusively to cover *all forms of grains, starches, and sugars* that promote weight gain, addictive eating patterns, and health threats. It's just like, on the highway, when you first near an upcoming exit, the signs will announce that you can find food, gas, and/or lodging at the exit, but as you actually approach the exit, only the exit number will be posted. In just the same way, when you take the *No-Grain* exit off the super highway of weight gain, obesity, and an array of health problems, you'll leave behind all detrimental carb foods, whether they come from grains, grain products, starchy vegetables, sweets, or desserts. So follow the *No-Grain* sign to health!

My program comes complete with:

The No-Grain Food Plan: A twenty-first-century diet in which you'll learn how to eat healthy foods amply while burning off poundage.

The No-Grain Recipe and Menu Directory: Gourmet dishes and meals that satisfy your taste buds and nourish your cells. In compiling these recipes, I've incorporated a wide range of meat and vegetable dishes from all ethnic and healing food sources.

The "Cravings Eraser": A mind-body toolbox (cited throughout as EFT) that will include instructions on how to:

Conquer grain and sugar cravings
Eliminate the emotional causes of overeating
Banish the post-diet "yo-yo" effect that puts the weight back on

But How Is This Different from Atkins?

Dr. Robert Atkins, whose diet was first introduced back in 1972, deserves the credit for his tremendous efforts in bringing the low-carb diet into the national spotlight. But just as the Atkins program built upon and improved previous dietary wisdom, the *No-Grain Diet* improves upon Atkins by overcoming certain built-in weaknesses in Atkins's plan, which impede your ability to lose weight and keep it off in a healthy sustainable fashion.

I provide a solution to the excess animal protein consumption featured on the Atkins's diet, which is cause for concern because:

- Hormones given to meat and dairy cattle create a surplus of estrogens in humans—*and my meat recommendations eliminate this concern.*
- Antibiotics in animal feed contribute to antibiotic resistance in people—*and my emphasis on grass-fed and organic meat and dairy sources eliminates this concern.*
- Animal protein can over-acidify the body, causing bone demineralization and bone loss—*while on my diet ample portions of raw and cooked vegetables will alkalinize bodily tissues.*

My improved diet strategy addresses all these concerns while incorporating a wider range of healthier foods than Atkins or his successors. I include organic foods, more vegetables, and international spa cuisine recipes, as well as the most necessary supplements and proven mind-body tools to beat cravings for grains and sugars. Here you'll learn the way to optimize your diet, using the best recipes for raw salads, soups and juices, delicately seasoned vegetable and protein stir-fries and curries, savory breakfasts, gourmet meat dishes like grass-fed beef burgers, and grain-free desserts! In addition, I'll guide you in selecting the right proteins for you. Not all proteins are created equal, and customizing your protein sources is one key to successful weight loss long term.

Why Most Diets Fail

The vast majority of diets fail due to cravings for grains and sugars, which are symptomatic of grain addiction. Let's face it, no one's addicted to spinach, or other healthy greens, which contain complex carbs. But lots of people fall off their diets reaching for breads, pizza, or cookies. When *Dr. Atkins' Diet Revolution* originally promoted a re-duced carb diet, many people labeled all carbs as bad. The best-selling book *The Carbohydrate Addict's Diet* first drew national attention to the prevalence of carb addiction and its attendant health dangers. But de-spite their astute diagnosis, which rang true for millions of readers, Drs. Heller and Heller's food plan was ineffective. Why? Because they allowed dieters to eat ample quantities of grains, starchy foods, and sweets for a brief period every day.

It's as Easy as Erasing the Old Tapes

Diets fail because after the diet, you return to your old habits. It's not because you're weak-willed; it's because you do what your body *tells* you to do. Like sucking in your gut for a photo, you can stick to a strict deprivation diet for a short time. But you just can't do that for-ever.

Over 175 million Americans are classified as overweight (with a staggering 80 million of these classified as obese). Why? Because these folks did what their cells told them to do—they kept eating grains. Yet, with a new diet and new wiring, anyone can erase the old tapes and create a biological response that works in their favor.

As director of Illinois's Optimal Wellness Center, and founder and host of one of the world's most visited health websites, *www.mercola. com,* of which *www.nograindiet.com* is a part, I have cared for over fif-teen thousand patients at the Center and provide cutting edge health guidance and information to several million site visitors annually. Over a dozen years ago, I watched helplessly as one patient after another went through the frustrating cycle of diet followed by weight gain. Then with one patient, something clicked. Instead of urging her to try harder, or concluding that she had an obesity gene, or was otherwise doomed to dietary failure, I sought—and found—a way to change the *messages* that her body was sending. The grains and sugars that she was eating were actually programming her to crave and eat more fattening foods. As her self-esteem plummeted, mental messages reinforced this unhealthy eating pattern.

By reprogramming her body and mind with a new diet and new

messages, she was able to lose weight and keep it off permanently. I continued to use, refine, and modify this plan and found that it worked for over 85 percent of the people who tried it.

One Giant Step to Losing Weight

The cornerstone of the *No-Grain Diet* is one simple secret to effortless weight loss. Eliminating from your diet:

- Grains
- Starches
- Sweets

Period.

Cutting down on these foods, which most diets recommend, doesn't work because even the tiniest bite of a grain or sweet will trigger your body to crave more. On the *No-Grain Diet,* you're going to get serious about weight loss and take a giant step forward. For a certain time period, you will totally avoid eating grains and sugars in order to *change the messages your body sends you.*

The three components of my weight loss strategy constitute a total reprogramming of your system for permanent weight loss. Total systemic reprogramming on the *No-Grain Diet* will transform you from an overweight person who struggles unsuccessfully to lose weight to a slim person in control of food addictions and cravings—forever.

Here's how it works:

First: Once you start eating the recommended foods, your cells get this new message: release fat and burn it. *The end result: you lose weight.* (See Chapter Two to learn the biochemistry this program is built upon.)

Second: With the diet, you'll also learn to use EFT (a psychological acupressure technique) to curb any remaining grain and sugar cravings. Instead of telegraphing the urge to eat fattening foods, your cells will send you the message to eat nutrient-rich foods. *The end result: you'll permanently conquer food cravings and overcome grain and sugar addiction.* (See Chapters Three and Four to find out if you're a grain addict and how EFT can help you overcome it. In Chapters Nine and Ten, you'll learn how to use EFT for every kind of obstacle you'll face in weight loss.)

Third: Using EFT, you'll change your self-image. Instead of telling you that you'll always be fat and there's nothing you can do about it, your cells will tell you that you're slim and have the right to be. *The end result: you'll easily maintain your new, slimmer self.* (Chapter Eleven will help you reprogram yourself for successful weight loss, heightened self-confidence, and abundant energy.)

Debunking the Fad Diet Myths

Eliminating all grains, starches, and sweets (in the initial phase) is the first step in reorienting your body's signals to transform you from perennially overweight to slim-and-trim. You'll find it's easy to be amply nourished and enjoy delicious meals *without* these foods. "But aren't grains healthy?" most people ask. "The Food Pyramid says I should eat more servings of grains than any other category."

Let me address this two-part question.

Yes, if you are at your ideal weight, whole grains *can* be healthy. But if you're overweight, it's likely that they aren't healthy for *you*. What's more, you're probably eating processed breads, pastas, and cookies—rather than healthy grains like quinoa, teff, millet, buckwheat, and amaranth.

Further, the Food Pyramid guidelines are ineffective for weight loss. They are based on theories already disavowed by such prominent nutritional scientists as Dr. Walter Willett, chairman of the Department of Nutrition at Harvard. Among these discredited theories are:

- All fats are bad
- All complex carbohydrates are good
- All protein sources offer the same nutrition
- High quantities of dairy foods should be consumed

Further, the guidelines fail to distinguish between healthy fats, like omega-3 fats, and trans-fats, shown by many studies to cause disease. Nor do the guidelines address the interaction between grain consumption and insulin balance. Why are the guidelines at variance with the best current nutritional and medical science? It may perhaps be connected to the serious conflicts of interest found by recent U.S. Court rulings to affect six out of the eleven members of the advisory committee that composed the USDA Pyramid guidelines.

Beyond Good Intentions

Misconceptions about weight loss abound. If you've tried Weight-Watchers and other calorie-based diets, you may have found that it's nearly impossible to permanently lose weight and keep it off by simply restricting calories. Why? Because your cells are still programmed to crave grains, starches, and sweets. At the first opportunity, these cravings will overpower your calorie counting and good intentions.

Repeated and unsuccessful efforts to diet, no matter how well intentioned, affect you physiologically, emotionally, and mentally. Here's how:

Your Body

Your bodily systems are programmed to respond to certain cues by retaining fat to protect you from famine. When you drastically reduce your caloric intake, it may trigger this physiological response. The result? Your body *holds* fat. Low-calorie, high-carbohydrate diets generate a series of biochemical signals in your body that destabilize your metabolism. These signals make it *more* difficult to access and release stored body fat for energy use. The net result: you reach an impassable weight-loss plateau. Instead, your body rebounds, signaling you to eat starchy foods, and these cause you to gain back all the weight. That's how high-carb foods and diets trigger a biochemical *weight-gain* mechanism.

Your Feelings

Repeated, unsuccessful dieting sends you on a roller-coaster ride of up-and-down weight loss and gain. You briefly taste dietary success, inevitably followed by failure, and this failure actually programs your cells to repeat your failure the next time you diet. That's why it's so important to break the cycle.

Your Mood

Perpetual dieting destabilizes your self-esteem and self-image. To regain stability, you return to home base: *you* with an ever-increasing weight gain. To change that pattern, you must reprogram yourself to create a new home base: *you* at your healthy optimum weight.

While prevailing diets emphasize eliminating fats, and controlling portions or calories as key to weight loss, the obesity rates in America have continued to balloon along with our waistlines, clear proof that these theories haven't worked for the 80 million obese. In fact, recent studies indicate that our prevailing dietary wisdom could well be a prescription for *weight gain.* If you have been an unwitting participant in this dietary experiment, with its attendant health risks, which I'll delve into later in the book, I want to set you on a better course. But right now, let me emphasize one thing. If you are among the 33 percent of American women, or the 28 percent of American men, who are obese, it's critical for *your* health, vitality, and longevity that you escape the odds and the obesity epidemic. If you're ready to change your diet, your emotions, and your habits to maximize weight loss, you are ready for the *No-Grain Diet.*

Which Carbohydrates Are No-No's?

Complex carbohydrates, found in non-starchy vegetables, greens, and fruits, should be the core foods you eat. Simple carbohydrates, found in potatoes, corn, and all grains and grain products, baked goods and pasta, as well as sugars and most sweeteners, must be avoided—

even whole-grain ones. When I tell my patients to eliminate this latter category completely, I frequently hear protests. "Won't I be able to taste the cake at my son's wedding?" asked Emma, a toddler's young mother. She gained sixty pounds during her pregnancy and couldn't lose it.

"You mean I can't have a serving of Grandma's corn bread stuffing at Thanksgiving?" Roy, another of my patients, asked me.

Let me be clear: I would certainly hope that *in twenty-five years,* when Emma's two-year-old son takes a bride, she will be slim enough to enjoy a few morsels of cake.

On the other hand, since Thanksgiving was only a month away, I advised Roy to enjoy turkey with non-starchy vegetables on the side and forget the stuffing. By using EFT, described later in this book, he was able to control his cravings for Grandma's corn bread stuffing and stay with the program.

If you need to lose fifteen pounds to fit into last year's swimsuit, then this diet is for you! Anyone who is healthy, non-diabetic, and only modestly overweight, can easily reach their target weight, by following the Booster Food Plan, and move into Sustain, the maintenance phase of the diet, within a few weeks. However, if you have

- A weight gain 10 percent over your target weight,
- High blood pressure,
- High cholesterol, or
- Diabetes,

then it's likely that you'll need to follow the Core Food Plan until these health problems are improved, to undo the faulty wiring and stabilize your health.

Later on in this book, I'll provide more detailed guidelines. During the diet's maintenance phase, after anywhere from a few weeks to a few years, the majority of you can minimally and selectively reintroduce healthy grains, such as quinoa, teff, and millet. However, I must caution you that if you revert to foods like French fries, cookies, and cakes, then your weight and health problems will return along with them.

Angela's Story

My patient Angela, aged thirty-six, weighed forty-five pounds over her ideal weight of 125. The weight gain had crept up since her early twenties. She had outgrown several sizes of clothes, and was now into a baggy plus-size wardrobe. "With so many girls in belly-baring jeans, why should any man look at me?" she wailed during her initial office visit. While worried that she would follow her mother, grandmother, and other family members who took insulin shots for adult-onset diabetes, Angela, like other members of her Italian family, ate a lot of pasta, garlic bread, and other grain goodies, often downing her meal with a soda.

After explaining why this diet caused her weight gain and put her at risk for disease, I gave her guidelines for the *No-Grain Diet*. At first, Angela couldn't believe that she could lose weight, keep it off, and feel healthier on my plan, but she agreed to try it.

After the first few weeks, she had lost five pounds, and was surprised that she felt satisfied. Replacing her daily breakfast Danish with grilled tomatoes and poached eggs with hollandaise sauce, or a double portion of grilled turkey BLT (minus the bread) wasn't a hardship. She had enjoyed meals like the large tossed salad with sliced turkey at lunch, or the stir-fried vegetables with beef at dinner, but she feared a family celebration the following weekend. The abundant platters of lasagna and cannelloni were sure to trigger her lifelong grain addiction, and she doubted she could pass them by.

After I gave Angela the simple EFT instructions, she prepared for several days in advance of the get-together, and when the day came, she was able to enjoy the grilled fish, marinated peppers, and endive-radicchio salad without any hunger pangs. "I wasn't even tempted by Aunt Maria's garlic bread," she reported. Angela continued on the diet and lost all the weight she had gained. Two years later, she has kept the weight off, and at their upcoming wedding, she and her fiancé, Mike, will be serving a delicious rice pilaf to accompany the entrée of salmon and asparagus with hollandaise sauce. Even though Angela can now enjoy healthy grains occasionally, on that day, in her size eight low-backed gown, she expects to be too excited to eat much.

It's Time to Commit

Now that you understand why it's essential to eliminate grains, you are ready to start the diet. All I ask is that you adhere to it faithfully for the first seventy-two hours—that's three days. Compared with the various deprivations and weird fad diets that you've probably attempted, this is no hardship at all. Eating generous amounts of the vast array of healthy foods in my plan is doable on the first try for 85 percent of people.

The Three-Phase Diet Plan

Giving up grain-based comfort foods isn't easy at first, but you can depend on the Food Plan (along with recipes and menu plans) to nourish you, eliminate hunger, and reprogram your cells. With never a hunger pang in sight, the *No-Grain Diet* is more about what you *can* eat than what you can't. The recipes and menu plans make the diet easy and enjoyable. Eating ample portions of gourmet foods, like my *Italian Zucchini "Pasta" with Tomato/Meat Sauce* or my *No-Grain Pancakes,* will erase any sense of deprivation. What's more, every single day on the diet will bring you confidence as you realize that your weight is totally in your control.

If you secretly await the Sustain phase, intending to sneak pancakes, potato chips, cotton candy, or other grain and sugar favorites back into your diet, after a few weeks on the *No-Grain Diet,* you may find that these cravings have departed. As your body becomes better nourished, you will progressively lose interest in all of those foods. A year from now, if you *happen* to sample a former favorite, you may be shocked to discover that it no longer tastes good. Don't be surprised if you never again want to eat starches, sweets, and grains!

The Start-Up Phase (the first 3 days)

It only takes three days to go *No-Grain.* First, you determine (in Chapter Six) which of the three Food Plans is right for you: Booster, Core, or Advanced. Next, you stock your kitchen with foods from your approved food plan (detailed in Chapter Seven), study the menu plans (in Chapter Eight) and *No-Grain* recipes (in Chapter Twelve), and you're ready to start. You'll start the diet with frequent meals and snacks during Start-Up while using EFT (which you'll learn in Chapters 10 and 11) to undo cravings.

The Stabilize Phase (the next 50 days +)

After three days, you move on to Stabilize your weight loss and comfort on the *No-Grain Diet,* adding exercise, supplements, and positive lifestyle changes (detailed in Chapter Nine) to support your health and weight loss. You eat regular meals and snacks, while continuing to use EFT as needed to nip cravings or negative emotions prompting you to eat. Once you have achieved your target weight loss, and/or upgraded your health, you're ready to Sustain this program for a lifetime.

The Sustain Phase (lifelong)

During Sustain, you continue a healthy diet, transitioning gradually and safely back to a minimal consumption of healthful, selected grains, in a way that never jeopardizes your weight loss. At this phase of the diet, you'll be able to eat modest amounts of healthy whole grains, like millet and oats, nutritious starchy vegetables, such as carrots, yams, and squash, and delicious fruit-based desserts, like my *Fruit Crisp.* You'll find guidance for reintroducing these foods in Chapter Seven, with delicious recipes unique to this diet in Chapter Twelve. Plus, with EFT, you'll never have to worry about backsliding!

Harnessing Powerful Emotions

Nearly everyone who starts the *No-Grain Diet* begins with doubts that they can do it. So if you feel doubtful, welcome to the club. Doubts, fears, worries, or any other kind of emotion are never obstacles to your success on the *No-Grain Diet.* Unless a diet takes into account the range of emotions that every dieter feels, it is bound to fail.

I could create the best diet with the best recipes and menu plans—

and I have. But what good is that to you unless I also give you the tools to follow and stick to it? You can read about delicious recipes like my *Asian Chicken Salad,* but if, driven by cravings, you then devour half a pizza, have I really helped you? Your time might have been better spent watching a National Geographic special about a distant paradise you'll never visit.

I don't want weight loss to be that distant paradise. I want it to be your permanent home. Only by understanding how your body, mind, and emotions work together to make you crave fattening foods can we unlock the secret to permanent weight loss.

New research on ways to harness the connection between body and mind is revolutionizing health care—and it can revolutionize weight loss. Biochemistry, nerve drivers, hormonal messengers, and feelings are in a constant exchange and dance of mutual influence. Below is just one example of this two-way circuitry.

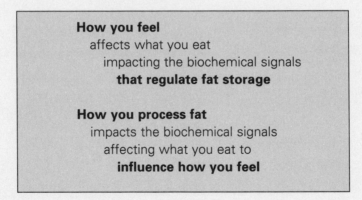

How you feel
affects what you eat
impacting the biochemical signals
that regulate fat storage

How you process fat
impacts the biochemical signals
affecting what you eat to
influence how you feel

Due to these interconnections and others like them, you get the best results by changing messages in both your body *and* your mind. That's what you'll learn to do on the *No-Grain Diet.* Instead of telling you what to eat and leaving you to face your struggle alone, I'll provide concrete tools to support your dietary and life transformation.

What to Expect

Diets lowering grain intake are not new. The first such diet on record was called *Letter on Corpulence Addressed to the Public.* Published in 1863, its author, William Banting, touted a diet that had helped him lose weight. It was widely copied—and attacked. This typical dietary prescription (over a century and a half old) has a strangely familiar ring: "One pound of beef or mutton or fish per day with a moderate amount of the non-starchy vegetables [tomatoes, lettuce, string beans, spinach, and such] will be found ample for any obese person of sedentary habits."

Yes, embarking on the *No-Grain Diet* will be a new experience, but one based on time-tested principles. If you are overweight, losing that excess weight is the best thing you can for do your health, now and in the long term. But as long as you stay locked in a negative carbohydrate cycle, you have little hope of becoming and maintaining a slimmer you. I'm here to tell you that can change. With your cooperation, I'll help you achieve the lasting success in dieting. Throughout this book, I'll coach you in going for the gold standard: total health and permanent weight loss.

CHAPTER 2

THE BIOCHEMISTRY OF WEIGHT LOSS

Before I ask you to give up grains, sweets, and starchy foods, I want you to grasp the sound physiological reasons why it's necessary. They may be called comfort foods, but the facts about their health effects aren't comforting at all. First, new medical findings confirm that most grains, not fats, are the chief culprits in weight gain. Next, study after study shows how grains and sugars take you down the road to disease, first causing metabolic slowdown, and weight gain, then leading to pre-diabetic conditions, diabetes, and subsequently to the three big killers: heart disease, cancer, and stroke. Even healthy people who don't need to lose weight, or who only need to lose a few pounds to look fit and trim, can protect themselves from a health downturn by going on the *No-Grain Diet*. What's more, this diet can help boost your energy and confidence as you take control of your weight and health.

Most critically, going *No-Grain* will safeguard you from making that destructive turn from grain consumption to grain addiction. If you are overweight and at risk, it's crucial to stop this health deterioration right away. Otherwise, as those pounds pile on, you head down the road to insulin resistance and Metabolic Syndrome (formerly called Syndrome X), which are precursors to diabetes. These conditions are all interconnected in a downward spiraling series of health problems. But the good news is that almost anyone can avoid and/or reverse them by following the *No-Grain Diet*.

Whenever my patients, or colleagues, question why I oppose excess grain consumption, I remind them that long ago in medical school, I used to be known as "Dr. Fiber," due to my enthusiasm for unrefined whole grains, like teff, amaranth, oats, and others. Yes, the fiber in healthy grains clearly benefits the body's circulatory and digestive systems. Unfortunately, Americans aren't consuming healthy grains. We are consuming unhealthy ones, including bakery items, bread, pasta, pizza, tortillas, breakfast cereals, waffles, pancakes, and fast foods. Eighty-five percent of the grains we consume are refined, the healthy fiber and nutrients stripped away before these foods ever reach our plates. Our bodies react to refined grain products very differently than they do to whole grains. All grains trigger an insulin reaction—and refined grains produce the most intense one. In fact, some argue that our bodies weren't ever designed to eat grains, especially in the quantities most of us do.

Are We Engineered for Grain Consumption?

Historically, the agricultural revolution was the foundation for our technological/industrial development. Approximately six thousand years ago, mankind transitioned from the traditional diet of the hunter-gatherer, which featured protein and fat from fish, shellfish, animal meat, animal organs, and/or dairy products, to a more grain-based diet. Was this a beneficial change? We like to think so. But some evidence suggests that it may have also had negative health impacts.

With ample fruits, vegetables, stone-ground whole-wheat bread, occasional meat and olive, safflower, flaxseed, and sesame oils, the ancient Egyptian diet was a modern nutritionist's heaven! Yet when studies compared thousands of Egyptian mummies to the remains of hunter-gatherer societies, they found that:

- Hunter-gatherers lived longer.
- Agriculturists had more infections and tooth decay.
- Heart disease and arteriosclerosis was more prevalent in mummies.
- Obesity, particularly abdominal obesity, was common among the Egyptians.

Nutritional anthropologists, compiling data from fossil records and other sources, found a significant body of scientific evidence supporting the hypothesis that genetically we are designed to fare better on the hunter-gatherer's diet—or a diet closer to it. According to their research, after grain consumption was widely adopted, the following negative consequences were observed:

- Decrease in height
- Increase in infant mortality
- Decrease in life span
- Increase in infectious diseases
- Increase in dental disease and tooth decay
- Increase in bone diseases like osteoporosis

In ancient times, the grains consumed were 100 percent organic and unrefined, yet still had these negative health impacts. Today 90 percent of our grains are highly processed, only making matters worse. Numerous studies of historical eating patterns show that our current level of refined carbohydrate consumption is unprecedented. Are our bodies designed to process the volume of grain and sugar carbohydrates with which we bombard them with in modern diets?

Loren Cordain, Ph.D., professor at the Department of Health and Exercise Science at Colorado State University, asserts that "Our genetic makeup is still that of a Paleolithic hunter-gatherer, a species whose nutritional requirements are optimally adapted to wild meats, fruits and vegetables—not to cereal grains. We have wandered down a path toward absolute dependence upon cereal grains . . . [and] it is critical that we fully understand the nutritional shortcomings of cereal grains."

Aren't Grains Healthy?

Carbohydrate foods do contain vital nutrients, but your body can make the simple sugars necessary for bodily functions from non-grain foods. Fiber and beneficial nutrients can better be obtained from vegetables. Grains contain little vitamin C, no vitamin A, and except for yellow corn, no beta-carotene. Although touted as good sources of B vitamins (except for vitamin B^{12}), two of the major B vitamin deficiency diseases, pellagra and beriberi, are almost exclusively associated with excessive grain consumption. B^6, which performs over one hundred functions in the body, is less easily absorbed from cereal grains than it is from animal products.

Cereal grains are poor sources of calcium, and if eaten to excess, grain calcium can displace more beneficial dairy and vegetable calcium. Further, with their low calcium-to-phosphorous ratio, cereal grains can negatively impact bone growth and metabolism by limiting calcium absorption, and by altering vitamin D metabolism.

Cereal-based diets (particularly if supplemented by vegetable oils) have a less than optimal omega 6:3 fat ratio, with deficiencies in the essential fatty acids EPA and DHA. You'll learn more about omega fats in Chapters Seven and Nine. For now, the bottom line is that some scientists argue that the human genetic constitution is better nourished by the fat ratios found in meat.

Glucose Overload

By far, one of the most critical problems with grain consumption is that grains elevate blood glucose levels, and thus trigger cravings for sweets. Americans consume dangerous quantities of sweets. Before 1900, sugar was a luxury item, enjoyed on special holidays and occasions. In the last hundred years, sugar (and sweetener) use has doubled. According to the USDA (the U.S. Department of Agriculture), between 1970 and 1993, the annual consumption of corn sugar alone increased from nineteen to seventy-nine pounds per person. For the last decade, overall sugar consumption rose nearly 1.7 percent a year. In 2002, the average American consumed a whopping 170 pounds of sugar, 20 percent of it in soda. And along with this expanding consumption, our waist sizes have grown proportionately!

Dietary Recommendations Gone Awry

As the consumption of grains, starches, and sweets skyrockets, our dietary recommendations have focused in an entirely different direction. Reducing fat intake has been the primary weight-loss treatment for the last twenty years.

Far from solving our weight problems, our obsession with eliminating fats has been disastrous. While carefully eating "fat-free," we've mindlessly increased grain consumption even though countless scientific studies reveal the connection between grain consumption and weight gain. In a study of three thousand people with type 1 diabetes, those on a low-grain diet had lower waist-to-hip ratios and waist circumferences (two key indicators for weight loss). Long-term animal studies show that starch-based diets promote weight gain, fat buildup, and higher concentrations of fat-producing enzymes. Yet despite all this evidence, grains account for 25 percent of the energy consumption in the United States. Between 1970 and 1993, the annual consumption of flour and cereal escalated from 135 pounds to 193 pounds per person. The average grain servings per day went from 5.9 (during 1989–1991) to 6.7 (in 1994–1996) according to the USDA.

Unfortunately, this astounding 14 percent rise in grain consumption was spurred by government recommendations. The USDA Food Pyramid urges us to consume six to eleven servings of grain a day. Currently, eating up to seven servings per day, a whopping two-thirds of us are overweight. If we continue to follow these misguided recommendations and consume the eleven daily servings now advised, it's likely that three-quarters of us will be overweight or obese. It's time to recognize these recommendations for what they are: a massive experiment that proves that consuming grain and sugar produces weight gain. Now that the results are in, if you have been a participant in this experiment, it's time to drop out, and take charge of your own health. And you can do it!

The Biochemistry Of Weight Gain

As you learn more about how and why the typical high-grain, low-fat diet is counterproductive to weight control, you will see why grain elimination is essential to reverse your weight gain and upgrade your health. Medical studies have confirmed that the key to successful weight loss is managing the carbohydrate-insulin-obesity connection—and that's the foundation for the *No-Grain Diet*. One study found that, after a high-grain meal, insulin levels were 53 percent greater than after a medium-carb meal, and 81 percent greater than after a low-carb meal. The authors concluded that a high-carb meal promotes excessive food intake in the obese. That's why successful weight loss is not about limiting calories but controlling insulin response. When you stop grains on the *No-Grain Diet,* you moderate the production of insulin, which causes weight gain. In a nutshell, even though carbohydrates themselves are fat-free, excess carbohydrates end up stored in your body as excess fat. This occurs in a three-step process, activated by the hormone insulin. I'll highlight the basic principles of how that works.

Step One

> Carbohydrate production stimulates insulin release, causing storage of carbs as fat.

Historically, the hormone insulin evolved as the body's mechanism to store excess carbohydrate calories as fat in case of future famine. That means that insulin aggressively promotes the accumulation of body fat. When you eat a low-glycemic (blood sugar–producing) food, like a chicken leg or a broccoli spear, blood glucose rises slowly and modestly. In contrast, when you eat a high-glycemic (blood sugar–producing) meal or snack, containing grains or sugars, like a bagel or ice cream, it generates a rapid and higher rise in blood glucose. To compensate, the pancreas secretes more insulin into the bloodstream to lower elevated blood glucose levels. Circulating insulin sends the message: "Store fat."

Once this disastrous scenario starts, you are in trouble. You will start to gain more fat; the fat will actually perpetuate the problem and worsen your insulin resistance by releasing free fatty acids into your blood, which in turn will further worsen insulin resistance.

Not only do increased insulin levels tell the body to store carbohydrates as fat, they also tell it not to release any stored fat. This blocks you from using your stored body fat to produce energy. The excess grains and sugars in your diet not only make you fat, but they make sure you stay fat. It's a double whammy, and it can be lethal. Instead of burning fat as fuel, which is optimal, your body stores fat. In order to release stored fats and make them available to produce energy, the insulin response must be moderated. The only way to do that is by avoiding grains, starches, and sweets, all the high-glycemic foods.

Step Two

> High insulin levels suppress glucagon and the human growth hormone.

Glucagon promotes the burning of fat and sugar. Growth hormone is used for muscle development and building new muscle mass. So if you want to become fat and flabby, you know what to do: eat grains and starches that cause your body to release more insulin, thereby blocking the release of these two key fat releasing hormones.

Step Three

> High insulin levels cause hunger.

Following a grain meal, insulin rises to lower blood sugar. This causes hunger soon after the meal. Cravings result, usually for sweets, leading you to snack—often on more grains and sweets. Not eating makes you feel ravenous, shaky, moody, and ready to "crash." This cycle becomes chronic. You never get rid of that extra stored fat, and your energy nose-dives.

This is called grain addiction. What you're eating drives you to eat more of the wrong foods. This is the biochemical reason why *all* starchy vegetables, grains, and sugars are addictive. Eating fewer calories from this category, as recommended in WeightWatchers and other calorie-based diets, doesn't work because you don't break out of the cycle of insulin rise, fat storage, and cravings. Instead, your blood sugar and insulin levels remain elevated, further decreasing your body's ability to burn fat.

Your Health Risks from Grain Consumption

How does eating the widely promulgated high-carbohydrate diet affect you over time? If you regularly consume grains, sweets, and starches, and avoid exercise, your weight will escalate while your insulin levels rise. As your tissues become progressively more tolerant to higher levels of insulin, you may develop what is termed "insulin resistance," a condition where your tissues have absorbed all the insulin they can retain. The effect is somewhat similar to what occurs when your vision adapts after you enter a dark room. The single strongest factor to speed the aging process, excess insulin also:

- Increases your blood pressure
- Raises your cholesterol
- Shortens your life span
- Increases food cravings
- Stimulates cancer cell growth
- Increases osteoporosis
- Causes type 2 diabetes

This entire syndrome can frequently lead to diabetes, and it's no surprise that 17 million Americans, nearly 7.3 percent of our population, are diabetic, with an astounding 33 percent rise in the prevalence of the disease between 1990 and 1999. Shockingly, there was a 70 percent rise among those aged thirty to thirty-nine years. I believe that there are an additional 5 million more undiagnosed diabetics. An even greater number (some estimates are as high as 16 million) are pre-diabetic—that is to say, they are heading straight down the road to diabetes. The *No-Grain Diet* can often eliminate pre-diabetes; it can frequently reverse diabetes, and it can nearly always reduce the need for insulin. For anyone on this insulin-related dietary downturn, the *No-Grain Diet* can be an authentic lifesaver.

The health problems created by excess grain consumption don't end there. Both obesity and insulin resistance accelerate your risk of heart disease. Diets high in grains also reduce the levels of helpful antioxidants, such as lycopene and vitamin E, which both protect against a variety of chronic diseases. In addition, since insulin resistance and insulinlike growth factors have been implicated in colon, breast, and prostate cancers, a diet low in grains, starches, and sweets may help you prevent these and other forms of cancer.

Osteoporosis

To maintain bone health, I advise all my patients to avoid sugar and high-starch foods that produce an acid pH in the blood, leading to bone loss. Increasing your vegetable intake, as advised on this diet, will help to balance your pH and safeguard your bones.

Autoimmune Disease

Many holistic doctors now believe that grains contribute to autoimmune disease, which occurs when your immune system, designed to react to cells it considers potentially harmful invaders, instead misinterprets the cellular signals and reacts to your own bodily cells as if they too were harmful. Viral and bacterial proteins are known to stimulate this reaction, and now an emerging body of literature suggests that dietary components—including those found in cereal grains—also activate this undesirable response. As a result, after eliminating grains, many of my patients with rheumatoid arthritis, MS, underactive thyroid, or skin rashes have resolved their ailments.

Celiac Disease

Certain grains, including wheat, barley, rye, oats, kamut, triticale, and spelt, contain a protein called gluten that is hard for many people to digest. If you have symptoms such as severe diarrhea, weight loss and/or malabsorption, or trouble digesting food, it's possible that you may have celiac disease. Milder forms of celiac disease, referred to as "gluten sensitivity," affect about 15 percent of the population—close to 50 million Americans. Causing damage to a variety of tissues, body organs and systems, gluten sensitivity can lead to a wide variety of common medical problems. Studies show that 5 percent of those with autoimmune thyroid disorders and diabetes have celiac disease.

Irritable Bowel Syndrome or Gluten Sensitivity?

Although gluten intolerance is often said to afflict one person in five thousand, newer diagnostic methods show that as many as one in thirty-three in the U.S. have this disease, which is often misdiagnosed as irritable bowel syndrome or lactose intolerance. In my practice, I've learned that it's very widespread, affecting as many as one in ten. Irritable bowel syndrome is often worsened by gluten consumption. I've seen many with IBS dramatically improve after reducing or eliminating their grain intake. It's amazing how often a wide variety of chronic health complaints clear up once people stop eating wheat, leading some clinicians to conjecture that gliaden, the protein in wheat, is indigestible.

A Diet Based on Biochemistry

To lose weight and turn around all of these negative health impacts, you will have to avoid all grains, especially for the first two phases of this diet, to allow your body to adjust to lower insulin levels. Once you have lost weight, you can move progressively into moderate whole-grain consumption, allowing your energy level and food cravings to guide you in determining exactly how many grains you can eat, if you can eat them at all.

Building upon the simple biochemistry you've just learned about, the *No-Grain Diet* will supply you with foods that correct the problem, and shield you from ones that cause it. Here's how:

1. By eliminating the intake of grains, starches, and sugars, you'll moderate the insulin response.

2. Increasing your intake of complex carbs from fiber-rich vegetables, while avoiding grains, starches, and sugars, will boost your body's fat-burning capacity.

3. Eating foods, like proteins and fats, that don't produce an elevated insulin response will help you feel nourished and satiated so that you're not tempted to indulge in the wrong foods.

4. Adding the right kinds of fats to the diet, you'll slow down carb digestion and absorption, further moderating the insulin reaction.

On this diet, your hormone response will normalize and your blood sugar, fat, and insulin levels will come back in balance, helping you to escape overweight and its long-term health consequences. At this point, you might wonder how to eliminate grains without feeling hungry all the time. Once you try the diet, you'll discover that with frequent meals and snacks, created from abundant proteins, fats, and vegetables, you'll feel well fed and satisfied. Every feature of this diet provides optimal and efficient dietary fuel to give you unlimited energy.

Once you have stocked your kitchen with the right foods to balance your biochemistry, your only obstacle will be undoing your grain addiction. That addiction triggers cravings for foods you don't need or want for weight loss and health. But until you deal with that addiction, you'll be at its mercy. Now, at last, you'll have a chance to overcome it. With your biochemistry balanced, the emotional and mental signals that lock you into the weight-gain cycle can be targeted and addressed through EFT. In the next two chapters, you'll learn more about how to harness this total revolutionary program for weight loss and health. Based on sound scientific principles, this program really works.

So whether you need to lose a few pounds to look good in the skimpier dresses, shorts, and bathing suits of summer, or you want to turn around an ample weight gain with its attendant health problems, the *No-Grain Diet* delivers twenty-first-century weight loss science in a way that's easy to incorporate into your life. Yes, you can turn around grain addiction. Yes, you can regain your health. Yes, you can lose weight permanently by letting your biology work for you—rather than against you—as it will on the *No-Grain Diet*.

Four Essential Questions

1. I've heard that protein consumption is bad for me and might cause "ketosis." What is ketosis? Am I at risk for it on this diet?

Although they might help you lose weight, diets with unmoderated protein consumption, such as the Atkins Diet, can induce ketosis, a condition in which your body burns fat, producing a by-product called ketones. Caused when the body has exhausted its carbohydrate stores, ketosis is one of the body's last-ditch emergency responses, and can lead to muscle breakdown, nausea, dehydration, headaches, light-headedness, irritability, bad breath, and kidney problems. In pregnancy, ketosis may lead to fetal abnormality or death. For all of these reasons, I don't believe inducing it is healthy. On the *No-Grain Diet,* you'll be eating abundant *complex* carbohydrates, in the form of vegetables, which counteract ketosis by providing a source of carbohydrate fuel so your body won't need to burn fat exclusively for energy. It's a much safer and healthier way to lose weight.

2. Isn't it unhealthy to eat red meat? What if the red meat is not organic or grass-fed? Should I still consume it, or limit consumption?

Commercial beef-raising practices are a genuine concern. Cattle, shipped to feedlots, are given steroid hormones and antibiotics that transfer to the meat you eat. They are fed large amounts of grain (primarily corn), which affect them the same way a grain diet affects humans: it "fattens" them up. The grains also shut off the production of a fat-burning, muscle-building fat called CLA (conjugated linoleic acid).

Organic beef is preferable since, unlike commercial beef, it does not contain hormones, pesticides, and antibiotics. However, unless the cattle are grass-fed, their grain diet will transfer the negative insulin impacts to their human consumers. That's why I recommend grass-fed beef, and information on obtaining it is in the Resources section of this book.

On the other hand, for most people, I do consider even nonorganic meats preferable to grains in the diet. However, there is a caution: elevated bodily stores of iron (resulting from eating red meat) can lead to heart disease and cancer. While menstruating women benefit from this extra iron, for men and nonmenstruating women, meat consumption can raise your body's iron to unhealthy levels, particularly if you drink a lot of alcohol, or regularly take iron supplements.

To determine if you're at risk, consider testing your ferritin blood level, with more information provided in Chapter Five, on page 71. While I don't advise lowering your meat intake, you can very easily help your body rid itself of this mineral that can increase your risk of cancer and heart disease.

If you have an ethical aversion to beef, dislike it, or don't feel you digest it well, by all means avoid it. You'll find many other protein options in Chapter Seven.

3. Do saturated fats on this diet increase cholesterol and put me at risk for heart disease?

Although it's become common wisdom to connect dietary saturated fat and cholesterol with coronary heart disease, there is little evidence that a low-cholesterol diet reduces heart disease—or increases one's life span. The Framingham Heart Study, often cited as proof of the fat–cholesterol–heart disease connection, tracked the population of a small New England town over many years. Forty years later, the study director said that "In Framingham, Mass, the more saturated fat one ate, the more cholesterol one ate, the more calories one ate, the lower the person's serum cholesterol . . . We found that the people who ate the most cholesterol, ate the most saturated fat, ate the most calories, weighed the least and were the most physically active."

Systematic reviews of trials studying the connection between fat intake and heart disease contradict any link. Researchers claiming the validity of the diet-heart idea do so by excluding negative trial results from their analyses. After reviewing all the medical literature, Mary Enig, Ph.D., formerly with the Lipids Research Group in the University of Maryland's Department of Chemistry and Biochemistry, concluded that increased trans-fatty acids were more likely the culprit in cardio-vascular disease. Her meticulous investigations of twenty-one studies, including more than 150,000 participants, did not find a correlation between saturated fats and heart disease.

Even though Mediterranean societies eat diets high in saturated fats from lamb, sausage, and goat cheese, they have low rates of heart disease. A study of the long-lived inhabitants of Soviet Georgia revealed that those who ate meat highest in fat lived the longest. Since World War II, as the Japanese have increased dietary animal fat and protein, their life span has increased as well. A chorus of voices, including the American Cancer Society, the National Cancer Institute, and the Senate Committee on Nutrition and Human Needs, claims that animal fat is linked not only with heart disease but also with various cancers. Yet when researchers from the University of Maryland analyzed the data upon which these claims were based, they found that vegetable fat consumption was correlated with cancer and animal fat was not.

The real issue is the amount of fat you eat, and contrary to what you've heard, most vegetable oils are the problem, not the cure. Before 1900, there was little dietary use of vegetable oils. By 1970, consumption of fats and oils from vegetable seeds was fifty-three pounds per year. By 1996, consumption had increased to sixty-six pounds per year, representing more than 80 percent of the fats and oils in our diet. Currently, every year, the average American eats nearly forty pounds of fats that have never before been part of the human diet.

This happened because, in the 1950s, the edible oil industry mounted a massive campaign to increase sales by convincing the public to replace traditional dietary fats and oils such as coconut oil and butter with its new oils, including corn, peanut, safflower, soy, and others. By demonizing saturated fats, butter, beef, eggs, and cholesterol-containing foods, the industry reached its goals. According to the U.S. Department of Agriculture, in 1909 80 percent of fat in the American diet was from animals and 20 percent from vegetables, while in 1994 40 percent of fat was from animals and 60 percent from vegetables.

4. Are saturated fats truly as dangerous as we've been led to believe?

Absolutely not. Many saturated fats deliver outstanding health benefits. Coconut oil, for example, contains both antifungal and antimicrobial properties. Butter from free-range cows is rich in trace minerals, especially selenium, as well as all of the fat-soluble vitamins and beneficial fats (such as CLA) that protect against cancer and fungal infections.

In fact, the body needs saturated fats for numerous bodily functions including:

- Utilizing essential fatty acids
- Protecting the arteries
- Using calcium
- Stimulating the immune system
- Adding structural stability to the cell and intestinal wall

I realize that this is a complete reversal of the health wisdom millions have known and followed for decades. Given our current health crisis, I hold that a fresh look at the data is warranted. Reevaluating opens the door to new insights. The news that we've gotten it wrong may seem daunting, but consider this. Although the previous analysis of which food elements produce weight and which produce weight loss and health was wrong, we can correct the misinterpretation now. Truly, the bottom line is not what the studies say, but whether the *No-Grain Diet* will produce weight loss and health optimization for you, as it has for so many of my patients. Give it a try, and I'm sure that you'll find that it can!

CHAPTER 3

ARE YOU
A GRAIN ADDICT?

In the last chapter, you learned why grains, starches, and sugars aren't good for you. But let's face it: right now you're probably thinking, "Oh no, what about my morning English muffin, bagel, doughnut, whole-grain toast, cereal, rice cake, cookie . . . I can't give *that* up!" You probably believe you crave grains and starchy foods because you *like* them. The reality is that, if you're like most people I see, you crave grain and sugar "comfort" foods because you are *addicted* to them. The *No-Grain Diet* can help you overcome your addiction, but first you have to recognize that *it is an addiction.*

The Truth About Grain and Sugar Addiction

Despite all the advertising and the wide availability of grain products and sugars today, our bodies were not designed to eat these foods in the quantities that we now do. "Why are so many foods prepared from them?" patients ask. "Why are cattle fed grain rather than their traditional grass diet?" Grains are cheap to use for these purposes because *you and other taxpayers* subsidize grain agriculture to the tune of millions of dollars annually, while healthier foods go unsubsidized. Due to the powerful Grain Belt lobbyists on Capitol Hill, we don't really have a free market when it comes to grains. We are therefore bombarded with this cheap and less than optimal food.

Meanwhile, the U.S. Department of Agriculture Food Pyramid encourages people to consume six to eleven servings of grains per day. Some may question whether the Pyramid (created by a government organization, not health scientists) could be a product of lobbying efforts and special interests, rather than actual science. In any event, the effects of this economic and political phenomenon cascade down to you, the consumer, resulting in grain overconsumption and addiction.

It's hard to admit that something you regularly consume is harmful, or that you can't control your consumption. It's hard to believe that grains are detrimental when everyone around you indulges in them. In this chapter, we'll take a look at the mix of conditioning, biochemistry, social pressure, and emotion that join to create grain addiction. My self-help quiz, later in this chapter, will help you determine whether you're addicted or not. To free yourself, it's important to understand why—and when—you're most vulnerable to cave in to the addiction. Checklists later in this book will help you recognize the situations, times, or feelings when you risk succumbing to grain and sugar cravings. That way, you can do something about it.

Grain Fever

"If grains aren't good for me, why do I crave them?" people often ask. A healthy system, in balance with nature, seeks out foods that provide needed nutrients, just as in the wild, sick animals are attracted to plants with healing properties. However, when conditioned by advertising, habit, and peer pressure, your body can no longer recognize and supply the nutrients you need for sustenance.

Eating the foods you crave *seems* natural until you realize their cost to you and to your health. Craving a pile of pancakes doesn't mean your body needs them. At one time in your life you *learned* to like these and other starchy foods. That means that, given the chance, you can unlearn that craving and instead learn to like healthier foods.

Once, a group of teenagers traveled to a foreign land where their hosts served them a popular local dish. The mystified teens noticed that this so-called delicacy was greasy and soggy, burning hot to the touch, and unpleasantly coated with something chewy and stringy. The teens were very hungry, and trying to be polite, they made several attempts to taste this food, but all of them found it disgusting. No one could manage to swallow more than a bite or two.

Their hosts were baffled since in their country, the foul-tasting dish was considered a treat. The teenage visitors were Haitian refugees, accustomed to a diet of fish, rice, beans, fresh fruits, and vegetables. The "foreign delicacy" was pizza. Without the cultural programming to love it, the teens couldn't stomach it.

As this tale shows, all our tastes are learned and can be modified. When conditioning rather than nutritional value dictates your food choices, you begin a downward spiral of negative health consequences:

1. Your cells starve.
2. You expend digestive energy to process nutrient-poor foods, harvesting little in return.
3. Your bodily systems function below par.
4. Low energy, weight gain, exhaustion, digestive problems, and illness result.

If this gradual decline in health occurs over an extended time period, you may not even realize it's happening. The good news is that you can reverse many health conditions and upgrade your energy level dramatically with healthy foods on the *No-Grain Diet*.

Why Grains Are Not Natural

Beyond the nutritional deficiencies and weight gain associated with grain addiction, other health problems are common. You may be chronically exhausted, have minor aches and pains, and catch every cold and flu that comes along, a sign that your body is overtaxed and weakened. You may feel that you must eat bread, grain products, or desserts with every meal in order to feel satisfied, which shows that your system is not functioning optimally. Craving foods like macaroni and cheese, French fries, or other processed foods that lack vital nutrients indicates that your bodily functions may be out of balance. Eating in response to external cues ("I'm near my favorite restaurant"), rather than internal cues of hunger, shows that unhealthy eating habits may be locked into your mind-body system. If you crave certain foods for comfort, or eat them consistently ("I deserve a cookie at the end of the workday"), it can signify addiction. Take this quiz and find out the truth.

Am I a Grain Addict?

1. Do you eat foods like grains, grain products, starches, and sweets at every meal? 5 points

2. Does a meal feel "incomplete" without bread or a dessert? 5 points

3. Do you feel hungry within two hours after meals with grains, starches, and sweets? 10 points

4. Are there certain grain and sugar foods you "cannot give up"? 5 points

5. Do you have high blood pressure? 5 points

6. Do you have high cholesterol? 7 points

7. Do you have a family history of diabetes? 5 points

8. Do you have diabetes? 10 points

9. Are you more than fifteen pounds overweight? 5 points

10. Do you feel unsatisfied after you've eaten a meal? 3 points

11. Do you ever keep eating after you already feel full? 5 points

12. Do you suffer from energy crashes after meals? 5 points

13. Do you eat based on external cues (i.e. "I'm near my favorite restaurant") rather than internal hunger signals? 3 points

14. Do you crave grain and sugar foods for comfort? 3 points

15. Do you use food as a reward? 5 points

16. Do you use foods to change your mood? 5 points

Add up your score. If you scored below 15 points, congratulations, you are relatively free from grain addiction. Still, you can benefit from the diet to optimize function, and going *No-Grain* may be easy for you. If you scored between 15 and 40 points, then you are indeed addicted to grains, and need the total program to lose weight and restore function. If you scored above 40 points, you are seriously addicted, and may face some challenges in addressing your addiction. I urge you to work with all components of the *No-Grain* program to assure you go through the process smoothly and successfully. The good news is that once you have conquered your addiction, you can experience an amazing change in your weight and well-being.

How Did I Become an Addict?

It's hard to recognize that you have an addiction when the majority of people around you *share* it. When a widespread addiction is not socially acknowledged, the burden of overcoming it rests entirely on the individual. Being addicted to grains, starches, and sweets today is similar to what it must have been like for an alcoholic living in 1930s America. Like an alcoholic, a food addict tries to quietly avoid the addictive substance, but when the pressure becomes too great, willpower collapses. For the alcoholic, that means reaching for the bottle. If you are a food addict, that means reaching for a starchy comfort food or sweet. People whisper behind your back that you are weak-willed. In the end, you feel ashamed, helpless, and hopeless that you will ever lose the weight.

But my message to you is simply this: while it's up to you to make the change, you shouldn't blame yourself. Daily contact with bagel and doughnut shops, pizzerias, and fast-food joints has barraged you with endless temptations to indulge in fattening grain products. At social gatherings, your colleagues, friends, and relatives invite you to join them in eating these foods. You need *help* to withstand the doughnuts, bagels, pizza, pasta, and French fries constantly parading in your face.

Programmed to Fatten Up

If you feel overwhelmed by ads pressuring you to consume grains and sweets, you are not alone. The food industry spends an estimated $33 billion a year advertising high-grain foods. These ads powerfully condition you to do what the advertisers want: eat more grains, starches, and sweets.

It begins in childhood. Did you know that a child's weight increases with the number of hours that he or she spends watching television? Research at Johns Hopkins University School of Medicine, confirmed by experts at the Centers for Disease Control (CDC) and the National Institutes of Health, showed just that.

By high school graduation, many children will have spent more than *three years* watching television, much of it commercials. During Saturday cartoons alone, the number of ads mounted from 225 in 1987 to 997 in the mid-1990s. And guess what was being advertised? Over two-thirds of current ads are for high-grain, high-sugar junk foods. In its drive for commercial success, the food industry is not looking out for you or your children's health. That means that you have to do it!

So far, these ads have succeeded in escalating consumption of unhealthy grain and sugar foods. Sodas now account for more than a quarter of all drinks consumed in the United States. From 1970 to 1998, consumption rose from 22.2 to 56 gallons per person per year, with over 15 billion gallons sold in 2000. Today, the average toddler gets more sugar from soda, a nutritionally worthless food, than from cookies, candies, and ice cream combined. This pattern increases as kids grow, with 56 percent of eight-year-olds downing soft drinks daily, and a third of teenage boys drinking at least three cans per day.

What's more, soda is sold in 60 percent of all public and private middle schools and high schools nationwide, according to the National Soft Drink Association. A few schools are even giving away soft drinks to students who buy school lunches. So while you're going on the *No-Grain Diet,* do your kids a favor. Eliminate soda from your grocery list.

Not only do cultural forces urge you to eat grains, starches, and sweets, but ironically, when you get the courage to seek help, you may find that your doctor is at best ignorant, or at worst, unknowingly addicted as well. As a result, he or she may also encourage grain consumption, perhaps advising you to eat "unrefined whole grains." While this is good advice if you are not overweight, advising an obese person to eat "healthy grains" is like telling an alcoholic to have a light beer. It only provides license for wholesale indulgence in refined grain products. Physicians often urge that you use a little willpower and eat grains and sweets a bit less. But if you're addicted, that doesn't work.

When Gloria, aged fifty-nine, came to see me, she had three decades of dieting behind her, and fifty excess pounds expanding her belly and waistline. Gloria shared a common misunderstanding that foods like pasta, potatoes, and whole-grain bread are "health foods." Recently, she had been on a popular low-calorie diet, and when I asked how she liked it, she shared her enthusiasm. "If I eat a grapefruit for breakfast, I get to have wine with dinner and a quarter of a baked potato with margarine," she enthused. "How much weight have you lost?" I asked. "I gained eight pounds, and I can't understand it. I'm starving myself," Gloria told me.

Like many people I see, Gloria couldn't understand why a low-calorie, low-carb, low-fat diet wasn't working for her. Gloria had reduced her daily intake of grains, cutting down her breakfast of cereal and bagel to a slim slice of whole-wheat toast along with two scrambled eggs. Eating lesser portions of pasta, and skipping the garlic bread entirely, Gloria found that her diet still wasn't working. Plus, her food cravings were killing her. For every "good day," when Gloria dutifully nibbled on melba toast and carrot sticks for a snack, there was a "bad day." Then she devoured a serving of fast-food French fries to "reward" herself, rationalizing that she was maintaining her diet by eating the medium-sized portion instead of the super-sized one. Instead of Gloria gaining control over her cravings, they were controlling her. The bottom line? Gloria wasn't losing weight. Plus, Gloria knew as well I did that her deprivational "good days" were priming her for a big-time boomerang weight gain, as soon as she quit dieting.

Following a low-calorie and reduced-carbohydrate-gram diet had indoctrinated a false sense of security in Gloria. If she stayed within its parameters, she expected to get healthy and lose weight. But calculating carb content can be misleading. People tend to lump together simple and complex carbs. Simple carb foods, such as grains, starches, and sugars, and complex carb foods, like vegetables, act on your body differently. Eating grains and sugars stimulates the body to secrete insulin, causing a rapid rise (and eventual fall) of your blood sugar. In contrast, each bite of complex carb foods promotes blood sugar stability. So more important than counting carbs is eating the right ones, and eliminating the wrong ones, and that's just what you'll do on the *No-Grain Diet*.

Some authors recommend "cutting back" on simple carbs, but this advice is based upon several common myths I'll explore and explode throughout this chapter.

Myth #1: Eating excess calories and fats make you fat.

The truth: While excess calories and fat can contribute to weight gain, *excess grains and sugars* are the real key to fat. Your body has a limited capacity to store carbohydrates, so it converts them into bodily fat. Overeating grains and sugars blocks fats from being used for energy, increasing fat storage. Eating healthy complex carbs, proteins, and fats increase your sense of satisfaction, protecting you from overeating.

Myth #2: "Cutting down" on carbs helps weight loss.

The truth: Since grains, starches, and sweets are addictive, eating less of them is like consuming less heroin, or any other addictive substance. To overcome any addiction, you must, for a period of time, *completely avoid* the addictive substance. Any grains and sugars you eat will prompt you to eat even more. Even healthy whole grains are metabolized nearly as rapidly as refined grains, thus contributing to increased insulin levels.

The advice that a little grain and sugar consumption is okay is music to the addict's ears. But if you think you can kick the grain habit without going *No-Grain*, you are mistaken. Even though it's the only known way to conquer an addiction, many diets and doctors resist taking the bull by the horns and telling people to give up grains entirely. From years of medical practice, I've seen what happens when people try halfway measures such as *limiting* rather than *eliminating* grains.

Like Gloria, they inevitably backslide. It doesn't work. Acknowledging grain addiction works. Why? First, because it addresses the underlying *biochemistry of the addiction.* Second, because it removes the burden of guilt and self-blame you carry after years of unsuccessful dieting, and replaces it with a constructive approach to addiction-free weight loss.

Let's look at the biochemistry first.

Kicking the Grain and Sugar Habit

Grains and sugars, as you learned in the last chapter, are stored as fat, causing you to gain weight and increasing your risk for diabetes. All these impacts are due to the insulin cycle. The highs and lows of the insulin roller coaster are *aggravated* by grains, starches, and sweets. Those same ups and downs program you for grain addiction. Remember this law of physics: what goes up must come down. That blissed out "comfort food" feeling that Gloria got from her French fries doused in ketchup was actually a biochemical energy burst, created by the surge in her blood sugar caused by these fast-glucose-generating foods. But that energy boost dissolved as fast as it appeared. In the down—the energy depletion that inevitably followed—Gloria's body insisted that she restore that energy high. And how does the body communicate the demand for more energy? By sending internal signals that are experienced as hunger pangs, food cravings, and intense appetites. If she resists those urges, she will put herself into carb withdrawal, feeling low energy and a heightened awareness of any negative emotions she has been using comfort foods to "stuff."

This is a double whammy, and if, like Gloria, you are a grain addict, this is exactly what's going on in you. Your cravings and hunger pangs are your cells' cries for grains to restore your high. Your emotions are on edge when they are no longer soothed by a blanket of serotonin, a neurotransmitter, released by grain consumption, which induces relaxation and a state of well-being. Both of these factors will drive you to repeat your indulgence, in an attempt to balance your metabolism and emotions. If you succumb and eat that bagel, you will find temporary relief through another brief high. But inevitably a low will follow. Continuing to seesaw between the highs of consumption and the lows of withdrawal is not a long-term solution because it does not bring you into a state of balance.

What's more, if you allow this pattern of seesawing between highs and lows to continue, it will become programmed into your body's operating system. Once this occurs, a "small serving" of grains will act upon you in just the same way that a puff of a cigarette acts upon a smoker. Instead of "satisfying," it only stimulates the desire for more and more.

To break this addiction, you must do three things:

1. Admit you're an addict.
2. Learn to differentiate between simple and complex carbs.
3. Eliminate the former, emphasize the latter.
4. Get the right supports for going through grain withdrawal.

Light at the End of the Tunnel

Once you've admitted you're an addict, you're on your way. Now, you may wonder what it's like to go *No-Grain*. At first, withdrawal may bring up unfamiliar sensations, such as cravings, hunger pangs, or negative emotions. But ultimately, going completely off grains, starches, and sugars gives bodily cells a chance to recover and reset function. Once you have achieved your weight loss goals, and reset your insulin cycle, you can safely and gradually reintroduce healthy grains into your diet, and eat them in a controlled, and nonaddictive, way.

"Are all grains bad?" people often ask me. Certainly not. Certain grains and starchy foods are healthy for people who can eat them selectively and process them well. Is it ever possible to be satisfied with a small serving of brown rice or yellow squash? Yes. Once you've gone through the initial phases of the diet, eliminated your addiction, and stabilized your weight loss, you can go into Phase Three: the Sustain phase of this diet. During that phase, you will gradually reintroduce healthy grains, starches, fruits, and sweets in a way that does not overturn your weight loss. When you are at normal weight or underweight, and do not manifest the symptoms of addiction, modest to moderate amounts of the right grains and wholesome desserts, like fruit, *are* healthy. But if you are more than twenty pounds overweight or a grain addict, then you need to reset your metabolism through the *No-Grain Diet.*

Recording New Messages

Diets that restrict grain consumption have been around for over 150 years. But to help you, first of all the diet must be healthy, and second, *you have to be able to follow it.* Unless you've addressed your addiction, you won't be able to stay on such a diet and keep the weight off. But now you can.

**Myth #3: There is no way to control
grain and sugar cravings.**

The truth: After the three days of total grain elimination in Start-Up, most *physical* cravings stop. Any remaining cravings are *emotionally* based. Now there is a successful and proven tool that you can easily implement on your own called EFT—defined below and covered in detail later in this book—that can help you to eliminate cravings permanently.

Up until recently, no one knew how to break out of the grain addictive cycle. Without EFT, urging you to get off of grain was like telling an alcoholic to quit drinking without AA. EFT is the equivalent of AA for grain addiction. It can help you gain control over the critical levers for changing your wants from unhealthy to healthy ones. Those levers are your mind and emotions. Learning how to use them constructively is the best way to consistently make the right choices and permanently alter physical actions or habits that don't serve you.

With my total program, your cravings will no longer have the upper hand. Beginning today, you'll be able to choose healthier foods. Rather than succumbing to either external cues or internal pressures that prompt you to eat unwisely, you can address food addiction and erase cravings for foods that don't sustain you.

Say Goodbye to Food Cravings

In any addiction treatment program, the first step is *always* the hardest, and the most difficult part of the *No-Grain Diet* is facing up to your addiction. You have already begun that process.

After admitting that you're addicted, the second step is admitting that you are *powerless* over your addiction. That means that you could not, cannot, and will never be able to lose weight or stop eating grains by using willpower. And I will never ask you to. Instead, my overall strategy will support your mind and body in overcoming your addiction. All you have to do is believe that it might be possible. We're not talking absolute belief here, just "Maybe I'll try it."

Overcoming grain addiction involves two basic steps. First, for a time, as mentioned above, you must eliminate all grains, starches, and sweets from your diet, which is what you will do in the first two phases of the diet. Second, you must have an efficient way to address the cravings that will inevitably arise, because unless you do, you won't adhere to the food plan. Without the second step, the first step can't be done.

Just What Is EFT Anyway?

Addictions of any type are wired into your biological circuitry, impacting your physiology and emotions, interconnected via your central nervous system. To permanently conquer an addiction, it's not enough to remove the addictive substance. You must rewire the circuitry so that you no longer *crave* the addictive substance. Seeking something to help my patients do just that, I conducted a three-year search, learning every technique I could find, in order to identify the most effective one. And I learned a technique that is easy, powerful, and profoundly effective in ending addictive urges. Its called the Emotional Freedom Technique, or EFT. Developed by Gary Craig to actively reprogram the nervous and subtle energy system, EFT, a form of psychological acupressure, has two components:

- You learn to tap on a simple sequence of easily reachable acupuncture points on your face and upper body.

- At the same time, you mentally concentrate on a Key Phrase. Usually the statement refers to a craving you want to eliminate.

In the next chapter, I'll explain why EFT works, while in Part 3, you will learn how to use it. But for now, here's how one of my patients used EFT to take her first steps toward weight loss.

Andrea was sixty pounds overweight. She loved grain products, ate them regularly, and questioned whether this diet would work for her. Her doubts were holding her back from even beginning the diet. When Andrea confided, "I hate the idea of giving up grains," I suggested that she use EFT to help her overcome her reservations. At first, she was hesitant, since EFT seemed "strange," but once she tried it, she found it easy to learn.

Andrea tapped on the simple EFT acupressure points while saying that she "hated the idea of giving up grains." In doing this, she was first acknowledging her feelings, and then releasing their hold upon her. After just two rounds of tapping, which took less than five minutes, Andrea suddenly began to feel that "giving up grains no longer seems impossible." After using EFT to help her take her first baby step on the diet, Andrea felt a ray of hope. She continued to use EFT and went on to a successful and permanent weight loss.

EFT is astounding in its effects. Even though it's new and unfamiliar, so were many things we now use routinely and find helpful, such as the toothbrush or treadmill when they were first introduced. That's why I urge you to try it. The only thing you have to lose is the pounds that make it impossible for you to wear that dress or those jeans you've always loved. With EFT, many people discover a rapid freedom from intractable cravings, challenges, and issues. At other times, a little more work is required. But it always promotes the healing process. On the diet, EFT will be one of your most important supports. Most people only need it for the first few weeks of the program, although some like to use it on an ongoing basis. With EFT and the complete and painless program offered in the *No-Grain Diet*, you can conquer cravings, undo unhealthy food conditioning, end grain addiction, and lose weight permanently. The many patients who've successfully met all these goals always tell me, "You know, Dr. Mercola, it was easier than I thought."

Unlike other weight-loss plans that you leave behind once you've "gone off" the diet, the *No-Grain Diet* is a *permanent* lifestyle change. By using EFT to handle the life changes that result from your weight loss, you'll successfully maintain it. Turning to EFT will protect you against temptations to backslide now or in the future.

The art of using EFT is how you create what you say while tapping. You'll learn how to input data that reflects what you feel and that works for you. I'll provide many examples you can use or adapt. You'll access real-life stories that show how to work with common issues in an ongoing EFT process. I'll help you address both simple cravings for unhealthy foods, as well as the underlying emotional issues that unconsciously motivate eating and weight gain. I'll offer strategies for using EFT to support your weight-loss maintenance program. By using EFT while on the *No-Grain Diet,* you'll permanently conquer grain addiction and move into a world of health, weight loss, and authentic nourishment.

CHAPTER 4

USING EFT TO OVERCOME GRAIN ADDICTION

Recording New Messages

Low-carb diets have been around for decades, but on other low-carb diets, the sole barrier between you and the wrong foods is *gram count*. These diets recommend that you calculate each carbohydrate food's gram count in order to stay below a certain number every day. If you do, weight loss is assured, proponents of these diets proclaim.

But that's a big *if*. While knowing a food's carbohydrate gram content can be valuable, counting grams is a cumbersome and incomplete measure of a food's effect on your body. What's more, it's not the best strategy for *permanent* weight loss. Here's why:

Theoretically, you could adhere to these diets by eating twenty M&Ms, which contain a slightly higher carb content than one cup of cooked broccoli. But practically, there's a big difference between the two foods. The M&Ms contain harmful dyes, fats, and sugars that will launch an insulin roller coaster, leading long-term to increased risk for serious and life-threatening diseases. The broccoli contains cancer-fighting nutrients, but that's not all. Broccoli *positively* impacts your ability to *maintain* your diet, by giving you a feeling of satiation that helps you to follow your Food Plan. Beyond their nutritional deficits, the M&Ms *negatively* impact your diet by causing a blood sugar spike that triggers you to eat *other* wrong foods. Plus, let's not kid ourselves, if you eat the M&Ms for "lunch," that's probably not all you'll be eating!

Now, I'm not saying that the Atkins (or other traditional low-carb diets) recommend that you eat M&Ms; obviously, a distinguished physician like Dr. Atkins advises *against* eating sweets and processed foods just as I do. I'm alerting you to the reality that often, when people try to live with a diet, they subtly twist it to suit their addictions. Just as on WeightWatchers people can choose to eat a five-hundred-calorie cake for "lunch," on Atkins, they may eat a "low-carb serving of" M&Ms or other undesirable foods, because, hey, it's only a few carb grams.

The real issue is not the gram count of each item but *how* you choose what to eat. If you had the power, you'd choose broccoli over M&Ms. However, despite broccoli's health benefits, gram count, and dietary impact, your body is deciding differently, and right now that decision is outside of your control. Why? Because your body-mind messaging center takes in all this information, boils it down, and then registers it as "I *should* eat the broccoli" but "I *want* to eat the M&Ms."

Practically, that means that you'll follow the "shoulds" for just so long, before your "wants" move you toward the wrong foods. No carb-gram or calorie counter can stop that inevitable slide back into wrong eating patterns, because they are all just more "shoulds." But starting today, that is going to change, as you gain control over the critical levers for shifting your wants from unhealthy to healthy ones. Those levers are your mind and emotions. Learning how to use them constructively is the best way to consistently make the right choices and permanently alter physical actions or habits that don't serve you.

Twenty-First-Century Mind-Body Healing

Your body, mind, and emotions are not separate, independently functioning entities. They are interconnected within you. In fact, they *are* you! As scientists begin to understand and explore this basic truth, let me assure you that harnessing all three levels of yourself is key to successful weight loss.

Right now, let's review how the three levels of your being are currently working against you:

On the emotional level: Negative emotions or memories prompt your taste buds to crave fattening grains and sugars and to eat them addictively.

On the metabolic level: Overwhelmed by an excess of grains and sugars, your digestion and metabolism tell your body to store fat.

On the mental level: Your thoughts and beliefs tell you that you are an overweight person and that it's impossible to permanently lose weight.

But starting today, you have the power to turn all that around. The *No-Grain Diet* will give you concrete tools to make all three levels *work for you.* Here's how:

For the metabolic level: The Food Plan (see Part 2) will permanently change what you eat and how your body metabolizes food.

For the emotional level: EFT will help you deal with cravings and negative emotions prompting you to eat.

For the mental level: EFT will undo beliefs causing you to fail and program you for success in weight loss.

The bottom line is: if you're overweight, it's due not only to *what* you eat, it's equally due to *why* you eat it. If you don't change the *why,* over the long term, you won't successfully modify the *what.* Traditional diets offer you gram counting and abstinence. But exhortations like "Remember that addictions can be managed only through abstinence," as the Atkins website reminds dieters, are just enforcing the *what.*

We'll take a step beyond that into twenty-first-century nutritional technology, by using your emotions and mind as levers to change the *why.* Here's how: to address negative emotions and beliefs prompting you to eat, I'll teach you to erase the old tapes that send destructive signals to your operating system, such as "I crave a triple serving of waffles." You'll also learn to record constructive ones, like "I lose weight effortlessly." To do both, you'll master the body-mind tool called Emotional Freedom Technique.

EFT has been used successfully by tens of thousands of people seeking weight loss, and emotional and physical well-being. If you, like my patients, are trapped in an unending cycle of weight loss and gain, with EFT, you can overcome the patterns that interfere with your diet, accessing your total being to create a *new* dietary outcome. I call it a "Cravings Eraser," because I've never encountered a more effective tool for ending cravings permanently.

EFT: A Life-Changing Tool

EFT is the most widely used form of psychological acupressure, a powerful new transformational technology that is changing the way we understand healing. I've been fortunate to work closely with EFT founder Gary Craig in my creation of the EFT applications for health and weight loss you'll learn as part of the *No-Grain Diet*. Currently in use in a wide variety of health and counseling settings, for everything from addiction to abuse to marital counseling, EFT actively reprograms the nervous system in two simultaneous steps:

You tap on a simple sequence of nine acupuncture points on your body. At the same time, you mentally concentrate on a Key Phrase. Usually this phrase expresses something you want to eliminate, such as a craving, negative emotion, or belief.

EFT can also be used to install a positive feeling, intention, or goal. The transformation that comes from EFT seems miraculous when compared with the slower timing and ineffectiveness of other methods in dealing with intractable problems. Plus, it's free, portable, and adaptable to your needs.

Case Study

Paula, a thirty-three-year-old administrative assistant, had uncontrollable sugar and chocolate cravings that resulted in her gaining fifty pounds over her optimal weight. She suffered extreme sugar cravings three to four times per day, which were particularly strong after each meal. On her first office visit I taught her EFT. Paula found the tapping a bit strange at first but she persisted, and tapped regularly for one month before and after meals. After just one month, Paula's cravings subsided so that she didn't need to do EFT regularly anymore. She still uses it when cravings reappear, which doesn't happen more than a few times each month.

"Without the EFT, I know I would have sabotaged myself and gained all the weight back," Paula told me. EFT also helped her deal with on-the-job stress. Whenever she faces a challenge at work, Paula goes into the bathroom to do her EFT. Recently, at her one-year follow-up office visit, Paula told me that she no longer needs to use EFT to control her eating because her weight loss is completely under her control. Instead, she now uses it only for stress, but even that need has subsided to a monthly EFT touch-up. Also, Paula was delighted to report that, in addition to losing the excess fifty pounds, the allergies and asthma she'd experienced since girlhood have also disappeared.

How EFT Works

For over five millennia, traditional Chinese doctors have inserted needles into acupuncture points to help move subtle energy through the body via pathways they call meridians. Meridians connect to all our nerves, organs, and systems, delivering a flow of energy to help balance their functioning. A blockage in a meridian pathway can cause an imbalance, and acupuncture (or acupressure) works by releasing that blockage.

Recently, researchers have learned that *tapping* on these very same acupuncture/acupressure points has the same effect: it releases blockages and sends energy to the corresponding system to optimize function. And tapping can be done by anyone, requiring no special expertise.

A craving, negative emotion or belief acts like a blockage to the flow of life force along the meridian pathways within you. When you tap on the acupressure points, and say the Key Phrase, it dissolves that blockage. It's like pressing the DELETE button on your computer—and then rebooting. You've erased the phrase, and your system is no longer programmed to act on it.

As an example, let's say that you love grain products and question whether this diet will work for you. You might choose the phrase "I hate the idea of giving up grains." As you tap, while saying the phrase, you first acknowledge your feelings and then release their hold upon you.

Dealings with Feelings

"What if I don't want to give up my feelings, Dr. Mercola?" some people ask. Rest assured that you'll be the one and only judge of which feelings enrich your life, and which ones hamper it. Feelings are fine, but do you have your feelings or do they have you? When nonconstructive beliefs like "I'm fat and I always will be," or feelings like "I won't feel satisfied without a second serving of lasagna" *have you*, they can sabotage your every effort to lose weight. Fortunately, thanks to EFT, you can help repair the short-circuiting they cause, rewiring your body and mind to serve you and your weight loss goals.

Modern science now confirms that emotions are experienced and stored in the body. In traditional Chinese medicine, physicians correlate each of the emotions with a specific organ and meridian system. For example, worry is correlated with the stomach/spleen meridian, fear is associated with the kidney/bladder meridian, and sadness is correlated with the lung/large intestine meridian. When balanced energy flows through these meridians, you'll experience the positive side of each of these emotions, so that instead of worry, you'll feel confidence, or instead of fear, courage. However, when they are unbalanced due to blockages, you'll experience negative emotions.

To bring an emotion back into balance, acupuncturists and other practitioners who use the meridian-based health model treat its corresponding meridian and organ. EFT is unique in treating *all* of the emotions, organs, and meridians to correct *any* potential dysfunction. Since strong emotions like sadness, anger, fear, or worry are interrelated, treating them all makes sense. The points you will learn to tap on in the simple EFT sequence delineated in Chapter Ten activate and balance *every* meridian in your body. You don't have to figure it out, you just have to do the same basic sequence for total healing.

A New Theory

Scientists studying brain function have given us a different theory for understanding how EFT works to heal emotions. Painful emotional experiences, stored long-term in a primitive part of the brain called the limbic system, disrupt your body's electrical functioning, negatively impacting your health and well-being, some advanced thinkers assert. How does EFT change that? Tapping on the acupoints on your head and chest opens up access to the limbic portion of your brain. As you concentrate on every detail of the painful emotion, event, belief, or craving, you activate and reprogram the brain circuits that caused the energy disruption. Gary Craig is fond of saying, "All—not some, *all*—negative emotions, are due to disruptions in your bioenergy system."

A more detailed explanation of this mechanism comes from *Energy Medicine: The Scientific Basis* by James L. Oschman.

Every part of the body, including all of the molecules so thoroughly studied by modern science, as well as the acupuncture meridians of traditional East Asian or Oriental medicine, form a continuously interconnected semiconductor electronic network. Each component of the organism, even the smallest part, is immersed in, and generates, a constant stream of vibratory information. This is information about all of the activities taking place everywhere in the body.

Complete health corresponds to a *total interconnection* [italics mine] of this network. Accumulated physical and emotional trauma impairs these interconnections. When this happens, the body's defense and repair systems become impaired and disease has a chance to take hold. EFT and other psychological acupressure therapies restore and balance the vibratory circuitry, with obvious and profound benefits. The body's defense and repair systems are able to repair themselves.

Many individuals, both scientists and therapists, have contributed valuable insights to this emerging picture of how the body functions in health and disease. Phenomena that previously seemed disconnected and unrelated are now complementing one another, giving us a more complete understanding than we could have obtained by a single approach.

I am deeply excited about these new developments, and have seen their phenomenal impacts on hundreds of patients. I know from first-hand experience that, by using EFT, you too can optimize your health and go way beyond your current health horizons.

Inputting the New Data

In Chapter Ten, you'll learn my simplified version of the basic EFT Tapping Menu originally developed by EFT founder Gary Craig. The technique itself is simple. It takes less than five minutes to do, and I've never met anyone who couldn't readily learn it. It can be done in the midst of other activities. Even if you mix up the sequence or forget to tap some of the points, it still works.

While its real-life applications are countless, for my program you'll focus on using EFT to:

- Conquer cravings and simple carbohydrate addiction
- Address underlying emotions and beliefs that trigger overeating
- Adjust to your transformation from the overweight you to the slender you

The art of using EFT is in framing what you say while tapping. In Chapters Ten and Eleven, you'll learn how to input data that reflects what you feel and that works for you. I'll provide examples you can use or adapt. I'll present real-life stories that show how to work with common issues in an ongoing EFT process. I'll help you address both simple cravings for unhealthy foods, as well as the underlying emotional issues that unconsciously motivate eating and weight gain. I'll offer strategies for using EFT to support your weight loss maintenance program.

Passing a Krispy Kreme doughnut store on the way to work every day, Jill developed the habit of getting a doughnut, or two. Well past her ideal weight of 135, Jill was pushing 160. Her clothes didn't fit. Those daily doughnuts launched a metabolic slowdown and weight gain, with future health problems waiting in the wings.

To turn that around, Jill began the *No-Grain Diet*. To combat her urges, whenever she approached the doughnut shop, she did EFT, tapping while thinking, "I completely love and accept myself even though I'm dying to eat that Krispy Kreme jelly doughnut." After three minutes of tapping, the craving was gone. Jill went on her way without entering the doughnut store. After one week on the Diet, Jill had lost five pounds, and never again experienced the doughnut craving.

Twelve weeks later, Jill had reached her weight-loss goal. Now, whenever she passed the doughnut shop, Jill was so busy talking with a new male admirer that she failed to notice the shop or the doughnuts that had formerly tempted her. Two years later, Jill attended a brunch where her one-time favorite, doughnuts, were served. Jill wasn't interested. Now into the Sustain phase of the plan, Jill was able to eat selected grain products. So she made the decision to try one small bite of the jelly doughnut, for old time's sake. "Dr. Mercola, I never would have believed it possible," she told me. "The doughnut tasted doughy and I couldn't even eat it. I don't know why I ever liked them at all."

Just as it did for Jill, EFT will take you beyond your food cravings—to a life where confidence, weight loss, and health are an ongoing reality.

Tap Your Way to Weight Loss

Let's take a closer look at the different ways that EFT can support your weight-loss efforts.

Cravings

You can use EFT on the spur of the moment whenever you experience a food craving. Or to eliminate a craving in advance, while tapping you can say something like "I'm afraid I'll be tempted by Cousin Betty's Angel Food Cake." It's also effective for chronic cravings, such as "I really miss eating English muffins for breakfast."

Once beyond cravings, you can choose to learn how to program yourself for healthy food choices, tapping as you say affirmations. But that is purely optional. For the vast majority of my patients, tapping for cravings alone creates success on the *No-Grain Diet*.

On the other hand, some people get excited as they experience how powerful EFT truly is. You, like them, may want to go one step further and use EFT to heal the underlying emotions that generate weight gain. For some, food cravings don't subside until they find the unresolved emotional issue triggering the craving.

Emotional Eating Triggers

Underneath food cravings lurk emotions that can directly prompt you to eat. If you're feeling sad, lonely, angry, worried, or in need of comfort, calm, sex, or stimulation, you may be driven to eat grains, sugar, or other unhealthy foods in an unsuccessful attempt to handle those feelings. Sometimes the feelings and food cravings are joined, as in "I'm unhappy about my . . . (job loss, relationship breakup, health problem) and want to reward myself with a . . . (candy bar, hot chocolate, apple pie)."

Whatever emotions arise, I'll show you how to use EFT to handle them, so that they don't overwhelm you, causing you to eat unwisely. Once again, this part of the process is optional. However, many people enjoy learning how to tune into their emotions, to identify what's upsetting them and release it through EFT.

Beliefs

After you've altered the cravings and emotions that prompt you to eat unhealthy foods, you can start to access the bedrock of negative beliefs about yourself that underlie these unhealthy patterns. Although at first you may not be aware of them, after a time you may notice beliefs like "There's not much I can do . . . ," "I don't want to rock the boat . . . ," or "You'll never be pretty like your sister. . . ." Such beliefs function as hidden agendas dictating how you think, feel, and act, often without your realizing it. For example, not wanting to "rock the boat" or challenge a family rule that "you'll never be pretty" could lead you to indulge in fattening foods that help fulfill that agenda. Until you uncover and transform that belief, it will undermine your weight-loss efforts.

At first, you may find it hard to believe that you have the power to change your beliefs since, by their very nature, beliefs like "Dad always said . . . ," "I read in *Newsweek* . . . ," "No one at work does that . . ." appear engraved in stone. Fortunately, they are not. Beliefs *can* change. What's more, *you* can take responsibility for your beliefs, and use EFT to actively change them, just as you undo cravings and negative emotions. Once you do, you'll discover that your experience about who you are and what you can accomplish will change, too. After eliminating limiting beliefs, there is nothing to stop you from losing weight permanently.

If you hold beliefs detrimental to your health and weight loss, I encourage you to follow the advice in Chapters Ten and Eleven to identify them and actively transform them, using EFT, one of the most powerful tools I've ever encountered for doing just that.

The New You

Finally, while you were overweight, your self-esteem and self-image took a real beating. Now that you are in the process of becoming slender (maybe for the first time in your life), your experience and beliefs about who you are and what you can do will be revolutionized. Losing more than thirty pounds will alter how you feel about yourself and how others see, respond to, and feel about you. If and when you feel overwhelmed by any aspect of this transition, you may be tempted to undo all your hard work by reaching for the wrong food. This happens because having the excess weight feels normal, both to you and to the people around you. Not wanting to rock the boat, you eat in order to go back to "normal." That's why I urge you to use EFT to change "normal" for you.

Unlike other weight-loss plans that you leave behind once you've "gone off" the diet, the *No-Grain Diet* is a permanent lifestyle change. By using EFT to handle the life changes that result from your weight loss, you'll successfully maintain it. Turning to EFT will protect you against temptations to backslide now or in the future.

How I Learned About EFT

Aware early on of the power of harnessing the mind, before finding EFT I studied and learned a wide range of transformational tools, searching for one that was simple and universally effective. Early on in my energy therapy journey, I studied TFT (Thought Field Therapy), a method created by Ph.D. psychologist Roger Callahan, which was helpful but too time-consuming for me to regularly use in the clinic.

EFT founder Gary Craig, an engineer, performance coach, and minister, also studied with Dr. Callahan, and became a master certified TFT practitioner. Later, Gary discovered that a radically simplified approach (easier for anyone to learn and use) achieved the same powerful results. And that's how EFT was born. In this book, you'll be using my own simplified version of EFT, which I developed after studying Gary's information. Today, according to Gary, EFT is the most widely used energy-psychology therapy, with many dozens of highly effective variants on the original. If you want to learn more about the fine art of truly mastering EFT, you can go to Gary's website, *www.emofree.com*, which also contains links to other variations. You will also find guidelines for finding an EFT practitioner in Appendix Two.

I have used EFT for the last two years with astounding results, and can attest that EFT is the most universally effective approach I've ever found. My patients use it regularly with great success, learning it easily in a matter of minutes. In Part Three of this book, I will teach you my simplified version of EFT, walking you through all the steps you'll need for your weight-loss efforts.

In the next section of this book, you will learn about the *what:* the Food Plans and Program that will give you permanent weight loss and freedom from grain addiction. EFT will be your incomparable ally in addressing the *why,* so that cravings, negative emotions, and beliefs no longer stop you from implementing the program. Now everything within you will line up to support your health and weight loss. Treating the total you, the double whammy of the *No-Grain Diet* and EFT will deliver results you've never before dreamed possible.

PART 2

THE NO-GRAIN DIET

CHAPTER 5

THREE DAYS TO GRAIN FREEDOM

Now you're ready for the *No-Grain Diet*. Giving up grain-based comfort foods will require some adjustment at first, but it's never been easier, because of all the supports you'll find on this program. In these next five chapters, I'll walk you through the diet so that you have everything you need to undertake it safely and successfully. In this chapter, you'll learn how easy it is to do this program, as I guide you step by step in how to start it and follow it all the way to your maintenance diet. Once you have read all the chapters in this section, and learned how to do EFT (in Part 3), return to this chapter to begin the *No-Grain Diet*.

The Three-Phase Diet Plan

There is tremendous freedom within the parameters of the diet. You should never feel hungry eating the healthy foods you'll find in Chapter Seven. You are to eat amply at meals and at snacks. If you notice that you feel hungry between meals, eat another snack of your allowed foods. What's more, you never have to count calories or carbohydrate grams; the diet fundamentals do all the work for you. When you eat the right foods, in the combination that feels satisfying to you, your hunger pangs will disappear. On this diet, you will get to know what works for you. And hey, if you eat a cup more Swiss chard than you should, you don't have to sweat it. Why? Because, like all the foods on this plan, that chard will never set off a dangerous insulin cycle, sending you boomeranging back into carbohydrate addiction. Choice and freedom lie ahead, once you become accustomed to this new way of eating. Follow a few simple rules, and you'll never go wrong.

First, **eat the allowed foods and only the allowed foods.** Instead of obsessively tracking grams, calories, or portion size, I encourage you to eat until you are satiated. I'd rather you ate oversized portions of cauliflower or spinach, or a second helping of halibut or broiled chicken, than a slice of pizza.

Second, **when you feel cravings for foods not on this plan, use EFT to erase them.** Note that I do not say "if you feel cravings . . . ," I say "when . . . ," because cravings are inevitable. On the *No-Grain Diet,* you have the tools to address them, using EFT. Now, for the first time ever, you can relax on a diet, because this diet is geared to your biochemistry *and* your emotional chemistry. That's how it delivers enduring results.

Third, **feel free to adjust your food combinations until you are satiated.** Because you are unique, so are your needs for proteins, fats, and vegetables. Experiment with eating more or less of any of the allowed foods to find the balance that leaves you feeling content.

Now that you understand the whys of *No-Grain,* you're ready to learn just *how* to undertake the Diet. To make it easier, I've designed the program in three phases—Start-Up, Stabilize, and Sustain—that will effortlessly get you into the program, give you ample time to lose weight, and move you forward into long-term maintenance at your own pace.

What's more, this program can be fine-tuned to your needs with modifications I offer to make it easier at the initial stages and more powerful as you move toward optimal health. In the next chapter, I'll explain that more fully. But first let's get a brief overview of the three-phase plan:

In Start-Up, you jump-start the diet with an introductory seventy-two hour program that eases you past hunger pangs as you transition into the diet.

On Day Four, you begin Stabilize, which includes implementing the full diet, exercise, supplement, and other recommendations. You stay on Stabilize as long as necessary. This allows ample time for weight loss, while giving your body and mind time to adapt and stabilize in this new healthier way to eat and function. Then, once you've met your weight loss and/or health goals, you'll be ready to move on to Sustain.

In Sustain, you maintain your gains as you transition into the ongoing nutritional program that you'll continue permanently. At this stage, you'll learn how to adjust your diet for the long term, and how to monitor yourself to *ensure* that you sustain the diet.

Before Starting the Diet

Set Your Goals

Before undertaking this diet, please set your weight loss and health goals. Knowing where you want to go is important. Next, I recommend you consult the menu plans (Chapter Eight) and recipes (Chapter Twelve) to plan your meals for the first week. Prepare a shopping list so that you have everything you need to begin. Plan both your meals and your snacks. It's most important to have some extra food on hand for additional snacks during Start-Up, if needed. Include some variety in your meals, but also have a few staple snacks at the ready for the times when hunger pangs hit.

In the event that you have a serious health condition, I advise that you more closely monitor your progress on the diet, in order to determine its impact on your condition. This can also provide guidance in timing your move from phase to phase. To help you do that, you will find more complete information on using standard medical testing with this program beginning on page 69. The tests I recommend can also be used by anyone seeking to optimize their health or validate the effects of this diet.

Get Real About Weight Loss

Weighing yourself regularly won't accurately measure how far you've traveled on the road to a slimmer you. That's because the permanent lifestyle changes made on this diet are not immediately translated into a dip on the bathroom scale. Reducing your body fat and increasing your muscle, as you'll be doing on this diet, is the authentic, permanent route to weight loss.

To track those real changes, I recommend that you measure your waist. While the BMI (body mass index) is often used to calculate normal vs. excessive weight, a recent study showed that waist circumference is more closely linked with cardiovascular disease. I also consider waist circumference a better measure because it reflects body density. Some people lose fat without actually losing much weight. You can tell if this is occurring by tracking your waist and hip measurements while you are on the *No-Grain Diet*. Fat loss is more critical than total weight loss. Weight trainers and professional football players, for example, would be considered overweight measuring their BMI, but at a healthy weight based on their waist circumference. What's more, it's easy to do.

Measuring Your Waist Circumference

Place a tape measure around the smallest area below your rib cage and above your belly button.

For Men
Ideal waist measurement: between 31 and 36 inches
Overweight: from 36 inches to 40 inches
Obese: over 40 inches

For Women
Ideal waist measurement: between 28 and 33 inches
Overweight: from 33 inches to 37 inches
Obese: over 37 inches

Another option is to use a pair of your pants as a gauge of your body fat. To do that, first find a relatively tight pair of pants to serve as your baseline. You know that tight pair of jeans? They'll do just fine. If you choose a looser pair, you won't be able to judge your progress. Use these pants to monitor your improvement. Your aim is for them to fit comfortably, or even loosely. As you progress, you can find another pair of a still smaller size. Now, with your weight loss and health goals in place, I'll guide you through the preparation for the Diet.

Managing Grain and Sugar Withdrawal

During the Start-Up, you will be going off grain, starch, and sugars. For many of you, this may be the first time you have ever spent several hours, let alone several days, without eating these food types.

> When it comes to treating an addiction, I have found that the only way to really beat it is to go cold turkey. Remember, the best way through is forward, and EFT can help.

Before you begin, it is essential that you make a menu of your first week of meals, and stock your kitchen in advance with all the foods you will need. If you fail to plan, you are planning to fail. This will launch you into the practice of sitting down once a week (at a time when you are well rested, fresh, and relaxed) to plan your meals for the week ahead. I have included a sample grocery list for your first shopping trip to ensure you get started the right way.

Sample Shopping List
For Start-Up on the Booster Food Plan (see p. 88)

Meat, Fish, Poultry (Organic and
   grass-fed preferred)
Beef, ground
Bison/Buffalo, ground
Chicken, whole and breast
Haddock
Ham
Lamb shoulder
Ostrich, ground
Shrimp
Turkey, breast or leg, and prepared
   sliced turkey bacon

Dairy Products (Organic preferred)
  Butter
  Cheese: goat, cheddar

Cream, heavy
Eggs
Feta
Tofu
Yogurt, plain whole milk, or goat

Vegetables (Organic preferred)
Asparagus
Broccoli
Cabbage
Cauliflower
Celery
Eggplant
Endive
Garlic
Green beans   *(continued)*

Vegetables (continued)
Kale
Kohlrabi
Lettuce, Boston, green leaf,
  mesclun, romaine
Mesclun mixed greens
Mushrooms, white and
  portobello
Onions
Radicchio
Red and yellow peppers
Red chard
Tomatoes
Turnips

Spices, Herbs, Condiments
Apple cider vinegar
Celtic salt
Chives
Cinnamon, ground
Coconut, unsweetened grated
Dill
Garlic powder
Ginger, ground or fresh root
Horseradish
Mustard powder
Nutmeg
Parsley
Sage
Thyme

Protein Powders
Choice of:
Whey protein
Rice protein

Fruit
Apples
Avocados
Cranberries
Grapefruit
Lemons
Oranges

Nuts, Seeds, Oils
Coconut oil, organic
Flaxseeds, raw, organic
Olive oil, organic, cold-pressed
Walnuts, raw, organic

Legumes (dried beans)
Lentils
Split peas

Miscellaneous
Almond butter
Anchovies
Chicken broth
Mayonnaise
Natural mustard
Wheat-free tamari soy sauce

Ten recipes is all that most families use routinely, so search in the recipe section of this book and identify ten recipes that you like. Ten recipes will give you the necessary variety, as it's essential to expand beyond two or three meals to avoid burning out and stopping the program. Variety is the key.

I advise starting the diet on a Friday so you have the weekend to adjust. For most people, the first day isn't too bad; by the second day, cravings or other uncomfortable sensations or emotions may begin to surface. With EFT, you will be prepared to deal with them so that they don't catch you off-guard.

Medical Testing

If you are a diabetic, diagnosed as pre-diabetic, or have a serious health condition, I advise medical testing before starting the Diet to establish a baseline. You can repeat these same tests as often as every four to twelve weeks during Stabilize to monitor your progress. When your test results have stabilized at desirable levels, this is one sign that you may soon be ready to move on to Sustain and the maintenance diet. However, I recommend that first you wait four weeks to fully stabilize your gains.

Blood Pressure

An ideal blood pressure is 120/80 without medication. If you're on medication, you may find that this diet will help to normalize your blood pressure. If after several months there is no improvement, please consult a health care professional who uses natural approaches, like EFT, to address emotional challenges, as underlying anxiety can elevate blood pressure. (See the Resources section for instructions on how to find EFT practitioners.)

High Cholesterol

In my twenty years of practicing medicine, I have seen over 95 percent of people with elevated cholesterol or triglyceride levels respond to the *No-Grain Diet*. However, people are often confused about their cholesterol levels, placing too much emphasis on their total cholesterol. A more important predictor of cardiovascular risk is the ratio of good cholesterol (HDL) to total cholesterol. Calculate this percentage by dividing the HDL by the total cholesterol (HDL/total cholesterol). This number should be above 24, ideally at 30 or higher, with levels below 10 indicating an imminent cardiovascular problem.

Conversely, if your clinician obtains this ratio by dividing the total cholesterol by the HDL (total cholesterol/HDL), then the lower the number the better, with a poor ratio indicated by any number greater than 4, with greater than 10 being serious. If you are one of the small subset of people born with a genetic condition called familial hyper-cholesterolemia, then this diet, although helpful, will likely not com-pletely normalize your cholesterol ratio. In that case, please consult a trained natural health care clinician to guide you in determining when to transition to the maintenance diet.

Insulin Levels

The latest figures show that in addition to the estimated 17 million Americans who have full-blown diabetes, at least an additional 16 mil-lion have "pre-diabetes." I recommend that anyone with any of the fol-lowing monitor their insulin levels:

- Weight gain above healthy levels (see earlier chart)
- High blood pressure
- Poor HDL/cholesterol ratio
- Type 2 Diabetes
- Serious health condition
- Family history of diabetes

In fact, to be on the safe side, I recommend that everyone do it. Here's how:

An economical fasting blood sugar test can be ordered by your health care professional from a reliable commercial laboratory, such as Quest Labs. A lab test is more accurate than one performed by your local hospital. While a home glucose monitor can provide a good ball-park figure, it measures a less accurate type of glucose. You will want as accurate a measurement as possible, since even a few points can be significant.

Type 2 Diabetes is formally diagnosed when your fasting blood sugar is above 126; pre-diabetes designates a blood sugar level between 110 and 125. If one of my patients gets anything above 100, I'm concerned, as I consider any triple-digit fasting blood sugar abnormal. A recent study by the Cleveland Clinic Department of Preventive Cardiology suggests that those with a fasting blood sugar above 90 are at a 300 per-cent increased risk for heart disease. Make 90 (or lower) your target!

You can also measure your fasting insulin level. Ignore the reference ranges from the lab, which are based on an "average" population that has abnormal insulin levels. The ideal fasting insulin level should be 5, and the lower the number the better. Fasting insulin levels above 10 suggest profound insulin disturbances. Levels above 20 occur in those who are actively diabetic.

When your insulin level is below 5, you can progress to the maintenance phase. Those aiming to optimize their health should aim for a result of <2, which you can achieve with significant cardiovascular exercise. This will increase the sensitivity of the insulin receptors, to radically lower your total insulin level.

Thyroid Testing

Although some doctors believe that an elevated TSH (thyroid stimulating hormone) level is the sole criteria for diagnosing hypothyroidism, I've treated thousands of patients who had impaired thyroid function even though their tests appeared normal. There are a number of tests that are more sensitive than TSH in determining if your thyroid gland is working. The Resources section reviews this complex subject in more detail.

Serum Ferritin

Since, according to many studies, excess iron can lead to cancer and heart disease, I recommend testing ferritin, a transport protein that shuttles iron throughout your body. With large amounts of meat in the diet, it's important to regularly take this test, which measures iron levels, particularly for men and nonmenstruating women. Fifty is an optimal level. Levels below 20 indicate iron deficiency, while levels 80 or above are elevated, and suggest iron overload.

Tests for Prevention

I feel that the above mentioned tests are important for anyone who wants to monitor their health, since obtaining a verified baseline is an invaluable tool for health assessment. It is routine for every patient who sets foot in my office. Why? Because I believe in practicing medicine preventively, which means catching problems before they occur. Too often, patients become motivated only once a disease has taken hold. These selected tests can help you find out your risk factors and use the *No-Grain Diet* to rebuild and maintain your health. While they are optimal, they are not a requirement, and those in good health with modest weight gain can use weight loss and well-being as their dietary parameters.

Checking In with Yourself

Prepared to address the symptoms of grain withdrawal, you're almost ready to begin. But first, tune into yourself and ask, "How am I feeling right now as I'm about to begin Start-Up?" Note whatever you feel. If your feelings are positive, anticipatory, or confident, congratulations! If not, turn to the EFT section of the book, and practice a round of EFT to address any worries you might have. Now you are ready to begin.

The Start-Up Phase: Primary Grain Elimination

First 72 Hours

In Start-Up, you eat every two hours to stabilize your blood sugar and minimize food cravings. On each of the first three days, you will eat three main meals and four snacks, or "mini-meals," per day. In addition to breakfast, lunch, and dinner, at each "mini-meal," I recommend eating a portion of protein—such as an egg, piece of chicken, turkey, fish, or some nuts—along with raw vegetables—such as celery stalks, sliced cucumber, or sliced red pepper. This combination will stabilize your blood sugar to prevent hypoglycemic reactions prompting you to eat the wrong foods. Chapters Eight and Twelve offer menu plans and recipes that you can use. There are also a wide variety of snack suggestions to prevent cravings between meals.

Here are the basic guidelines you will begin now and follow throughout all phases of the *No-Grain Diet*:

1. Eliminate all grains, grain products, sweeteners, and starchy vegetables, and food products made from them.

2. Choose foods from the Food Plan (detailed in Chapter Seven) and eat them every two hours until satisfied, to balance metabolic cycles and reduce cravings.

3. Use EFT (see Part 3: Overcoming Cravings) as needed to combat cravings, or other negative emotions or sensations.

4. Drink plenty of clean water. (See Chapter Nine for a more complete discussion of my recommendations on water consumption.)

5. Find your own personal fuel mix.

Here is a sample eating plan for the first three days of Start-Up on the Booster Food Plan; you'll learn more about the three different Food Plans—Booster, Core, and Advanced—in the next two chapters.

Booster Food Plan: Start-Up Sample Menu Plan			
	DAY 1	**DAY 2**	**DAY 3**
6 A.M. Snack	*Midsummer Gazpacho Energy Soup** Organic goat cheddar Sliced red pepper	*Baked Apple** with walnuts and organic goat yogurt	Grapefruit slices and turkey strips over greens with citrus dressing
8 A.M. Breakfast	*Mushroom-Chicken Quiche** with bacon	*Thai Sausage Patty** Cheese omelette with grilled tomatoes	*No-Grain Pancakes** with grilled turkey hash
10 A.M. Snack	Quick-garden green soup and crispy chicken wing or breast	*Creamy Broccoli Soup** and beef slices with horseradish sauce	Yellow pepper stuffed with walnut butter and chicken slices
Noon Lunch	*Asian Chicken Salad** on a bed of greens Steamed garlic green beans	Open-faced beef with *Gravy** over *No-Grain Bread** *Dilly Slaw**	*Tandoori Lamb Kabobs** with goat yogurt/cucumber salad Sautéed kale with grilled onions

(continued)

	DAY 1	DAY 2	DAY 3
2 P.M. Snack	Lentil soup with Swiss cheese topping and turkey bacon bits Raw cucumber slices	Radicchio-endive salad with goat cheese and mustard-pepper vinaigrette	*Creamy Fish Cake** over Boston lettuce with lemon-horseradish sauce
4 P.M. Snack	Cranberry protein smoothie	Walnut protein drink and *Beef Roll-Ups** with garlic dipping sauce	Grass-fed buffalo meatball "hero" served between grilled eggplant slices
6 P.M. Dinner	Grass-fed prime ribs of beef with Caesar salad and steamed buttered cauliflower	Greek lamb Moussaka Greek salad Steamed red chard	Baked creamed haddock over asparagus with mesclun salad
8 P.M. Snack	Celery stuffed with *Hummus** Grass-fed chunks of beef	Broiled baby portobellos stuffed with onions/lamb sauté	Pear with goat cheese

* Recipes can be found in Chapter Twelve.

This may seem like a lot of meals, but remember, you are reeducating your body biochemistry toward wholesome foods, and away from unhealthy and addictive ones. That's why it's essential that your cells receive ample nourishment during the critical Start-Up. Always eat until you feel satisfied, but not stuffed. Feel free to adjust the amounts at any of the meals or snacks, to find the right balance for you. If you're feeling full when snack time comes, taking just one small bite of your snack will ensure that you don't become hungry later and reach for a candy bar, power bar, soda, or other food not on this diet. Eating the right foods every two hours keeps your blood sugar levels steady.

Your Personal Fuel Mix

Food is made up of micronutrients: protein, fats, and carbohydrates. The body uses these nutrients to create energy, but the way *your* body does this is slightly different from anyone else's. The reason why some swear by one diet, while an opposing camp swear by its opposite, is that we are each metabolically unique. Some need more protein, some more carbs; people's abilities to process fats differ as well. You may have noticed that your spouse, child, friend, parent, or sibling has radically different food preferences. These preferences indicate the person's needs for nutrients. Some don't feel satisfied without ample quantities of heavier proteins, while others prefer lighter proteins with lots of vegetables. As a result of these individual metabolic needs, each person's correct fuel mix is also unique.

On this diet, I recommend that you monitor your energy levels to help you determine which mixture of foods gives *you* the most energy. There are tests that will actually determine your personal mix (see the Resources section), but you can learn to do it yourself. Here's how:

How to Find Your Personal Fuel Mix

Pick the same meal every day for your experiment in adjusting your protein-to-carb ratio.

- At lunch on Monday, eat your typical serving size of protein and vegetables.
- Tuesday lunch, eat a little more protein and a little less vegetables.
- Wednesday lunch, try a little less protein and a little more vegetables.

Pay attention to how you feel and function an hour after each meal. If you feel irritable, sluggish, wired, or experience cravings, then you haven't found your optimal mix. If you feel energized, optimistic, and alert, than you've found the key. Continue eating approximately these amounts at every meal and snack. It may surprise you to discover your true requirements. Once you do, you will experience an upsurge of health and energy when eating your correct fuel mix.

The Stabilize Phase: Permanent Grain Elimination

Days 4–50+

After the first seventy-two hours, you will pass automatically into Stabilize. Please check in with yourself at this transition, and see how you've fared so far. Noting your body-mind state throughout the Diet can serve as a benchmark for your progress. It also builds the practice of self-attunement that is key to proactively addressing the cravings and emotions fueling grain addiction.

Now that you have cleared the primary period of grain elimination, in Stabilize you can make these slight modifications:

- Continue to eliminate grains, starches, and sweets, and to eat only the allowed foods.
- Continue to use EFT as needed.
- Discontinue the practice of eating every two hours.
- Instead eat three moderate meals and three small snacks. You should eat one snack between breakfast and lunch, and one snack between lunch and dinner. If you eat an early dinner and feel that you need to, you can have an optional snack after dinner, but keep it small and light. In addition, do not eat for two hours prior to bedtime, to give your body ample opportunity to begin digesting your food before sleep.
- Add exercise five times per week. (See Chapter Nine.)
- Introduce recommended and optional supplements. (See Chapter Nine.)

In moving on from Start-Up to Stabilize, the only exception I make is for seriously ill people, who may prolong the amount of time they stay in Start-Up, if they find that the two-hour meal cycle helps them feel nourished. During Stabilize, you will eat the same exact Food Plan as you did in Start-Up.

> ### Moving from Start-Up to Stabilize
>
> The only difference is that instead of eating every two hours, you will eat four to six meals a day.

The menu plans in Chapter Eight show you a balanced diet. However, I encourage you to adjust it to your own needs. Consume sufficient protein and vegetables so that *you* feel satisfied after every meal or snack. If that means upping your intake of the recommended proteins, vegetables, and fats, do it. Likewise, if it means lowering them. Yes, you can feel free to eat more vegetables, and less protein, if that seems right to you. Your needs may shift over time, so retest your right fuel mix every so often. Let your sense of satiation, energy level, and mood be your guides. Remember you're unique, and you and you alone can judge the right fuel mix for you. The *No-Grain Diet* is not reliant on rigid percentages of carbs, proteins, and fat. If you eat from the approved food list, you cannot make a mistake.

Be a Nibbler, Not a Gorger

Certain of our biological ancestors, both human and animal, gorged themselves when food was available, to store fat for times of famine. But the very same biochemical mechanism that helped them to survive will shorten your life if you eat as they did, tucking into large meals while tightening your belt in between. Indeed, if you've tried this, you may notice that you need to add notches to your belt, because this is the ideal formula for escalating weight gain.

Let's face it, living in times of plenty, as we do, these bygone eating patterns no longer serve us. Instead, recent studies suggest that we should emulate those forebears, animal and human, who grazed, nibbling smaller quantities of food at many small meals. This eating style sends our cells the message that there's plenty of food. As a result, they release fat and cholesterol, lowering insulin levels and increasing insulin sensitivity—all triggers for weight loss. An added benefit, as one study found, is that eating more frequent, smaller meals lowers the risk of heart disease. Frequent meals also help your adrenal glands better regulate cortisol levels, to keep your energy even and reduce stress.

You may have noticed that most babies and small children naturally eat this way, grazing on a piece of fruit, eating a few spoonfuls of yogurt, or cereal, until they "learn" the correct way from adults. The more frequent meals on the *No-Grain Diet* actually restore you to a more natural and healthy way to eat.

If the Program Isn't Working

If you follow the Diet successfully and still don't achieve weight loss according to your goals, I recommend that you do the following:

- Move up a notch in your Food Plan. (Consult Chapters Six and Seven for more information on the three Food Plans.)
- Restrict your daily caloric consumption to one thousand calories per day, eating a diet high in fats. Similar to the Eskimo diet, you can eat five 200-calorie meals with 75 to 90 percent of the calories from fat. Designed for those with profound insulin resistance, this semi-fast effectively breaks that cycle. Most people don't experience much hunger.
- Increase the amount and intensity of your exercise, also incorporating strength training. (See Chapter Nine.)
- Go for thyroid testing to determine if you might benefit from short-term thyroid hormone replacement. (See the Resources section for instructions.)

Finally, if you've adhered strictly to the Diet for two to three weeks, have used EFT, and have tried all the above, and you still find you are not losing weight, don't lose hope. Since each one of us is unique, and therefore metabolizes nutrients differently, some people actually need a small and regulated amount of starchy vegetables and healthy grains to metabolize food efficiently and lose weight. In order to determine absolutely whether you are in that category, you may want to consult a nutritionist familiar with metabolic typing, a new form of nutritional diagnosis gaining popularity with many holistic doctors. You can find a referral on-line at *www.healthexcel.com* as well as more information in the Resources section.

Or to get a sense if you are in that group, take my Quick Metabolic Profile Quiz below.

Quick Metabolic Profile Quiz

1. At Thanksgiving, do you prefer:
   A. Dark meat (drumstick)
   B. White meat (breast)
2. How do you feel one half hour after a high-protein lunch or dinner on this diet?
   A. Satisfied, energized, and/or calm
   B. Cranky, tired, and/or craving something else to eat
3. If you believed them both to be equally healthy, which would you prefer?
   A. Steak
   B. Chicken breast
4. Which more closely captures how coffee affects you?
   A. Coffee makes me jittery and disrupts my sleep if I drink it too late in the day
   B. I can drink several cups a day and sleep at night

If you answered B to all four questions, it's possible that you may have attained all the benefits of total grain elimination and can now move on to Sustain. For your unique metabolism, you may *require* a regulated amount of healthy grains—in order to lose weight. Unlike the majority of people, who can subsist on protein, fats, and vegetables to achieve their weight-loss goals, you may need a small amount of healthy grains for optimal metabolic function, as indicated by your test responses. In Part 3, I'll explain further why factors like favored meat choices are important clues in optimizing your diet. In any case, to incorporate grains at this point, you'll find specific instructions in the Sustain guidelines below. Please follow them carefully, for if you do not reintroduce them in the graduated way recommended, you will lose all the benefits of the diet. If this applies to you, you may skip ahead to Sustain right now.

If, however, you answered A to more than half the questions, I recommend that you continue with grain abstinence, checking to make sure that you are strictly adhering to the diet. You can also go on the calorie-restricted diet as recommended above for several weeks to kick start your weight loss.

How Long Do I Stabilize?

I advise you to stay on Stabilize as long as necessary to achieve your weight-loss goals and/or to address specific health conditions that you have defined at the outset of the program. Measure your waist, or get out that pair of tight pants and use them to judge your progress. In addition, once you have achieved your goal, I want you to stay with Stabilize for anywhere from two to six weeks to begin a gentle transition into Sustain. Making the transition to maintenance is a big step. Your body needs to become accustomed to your new weight; your mind and emotions must ready you for the transition. You will use EFT to support you through that process.

If you have a more serious health condition, I advise that you move on to Sustain only when your health condition has stabilized for at least four weeks, as measured by the medical tests I recommended earlier in this chapter.

Successful Transition to Sustain

The transition from the initial weight loss to the maintenance phase of any diet is critical. That's where many popular diets, like Weight-Watchers or the Atkins Diet, fall. All the suppressed cravings, held in check for months, are right there boomeranging back with even greater urgency. Willpower, as I've said before, rarely works long-term. It's like holding your breath. You can do it only so long before you have to breathe out.

That rebound effect is nearly universal with conventional dieting.

And here is where the *No-Grain Diet* really pays off. Instead of using willpower to suppress cravings, you've already dealt with the underlying causes of weight gain and grain addiction. You've eliminated the cravings that tempt you to eat unhealthy foods. You've replaced them with satisfying nutrition, not temporarily but permanently. You've worked through your emotional obstacles to weight loss.

The Sustain Phase: Lifelong Health and Weight Loss

Days 50+

In Sustain, you continue the same diet with one difference. Now that you've met your weight-loss goals, you can gradually begin to reintroduce healthy grains. You will continue eating the same foods you enjoyed in Start-Up and Stabilize, except that for most of you, once your insulin cycle has returned to balance, it will be safe to gradually reincorporate healthy grains, starches, and fruits into your diet. However, I caution you to introduce them slowly and carefully, while following the Carb Quota Monitor outlined later in this chapter. Then, gradually increase your starch and grain servings to a one-half-cup serving size of foods from the allowed list. Continue to monitor your weight. If your weight increases or if you experience any of these symptoms, you will need to eliminate them again, perhaps permanently:

- Hunger
- Cravings for sweets
- Low energy
- Hyper energy
- Negative emotions, such as depression, anxiety, anger, irritability

However, for most people, once you have rebalanced your insulin metabolism, healthy grains and starches will convey some benefits. If you don't increase weight after a month, you can slowly increase your grain consumption, while continuing to monitor your weight. Proceed carefully as you reintroduce grains, as they may rekindle your grain addiction.

Allowed grains include:

- Quinoa
- Rice
- Millet
- Teff
- Oats
- Amaranth
- Buckwheat

I want to reemphasize that certain foods are still eliminated from the Sustain diet and, in my view, except for rare occasions, should be avoided permanently. These include such grain products as:

- Flours
- Pasta
- Cakes
- Crackers
- Sweets
- Sodas
- Anything containing artificial sweeteners

Please continue to avoid all trans-fats, as well. You will find these in margarine, all deep-fried foods, and in any baked products and pre-pared foods that contain partially hydrogenated vegetable oils.

If during grain reintroduction you find that your weight begins to creep back up, immediately halt the process, and continue on a pro-gram of minimal grain use for another few weeks, before testing again whether your body can handle it.

To learn how to reintroduce starches and grains safely, carefully fol-low the Carb Quota Monitor that I've included later in the chapter. Here are the foods you will reintroduce:

- First, root vegetables, like yams, squashes, artichokes, carrots, and beets
- Second, healthy grains from the approved list
- Third, fruits, such as apples, blueberries, grapefruit, and others on the approved food lists
- Fourth, healthy sweeteners (see approved choices in Chapter Seven)

The Carb Quota Monitor will help you determine the rate and level of starch, grain, and sweet consumption right for you. You begin on

Monday, and each day progressively add the food items in the precise amount listed in the Monitor. Remember that pair of pants you used as a body fat gauge? Now is the time to get them out, put them on, and check that your weight loss remains stable as you reintroduce grains. Check how the pants feel and how they look on you, as you continue to add foods each successive day, as shown in the Monitor. As soon as you notice that the pants feel the slightest bit tighter, stop! Do not continue to add foods. Instead, go back to the prior day and maintain the food amounts at which your weight loss remained stable. Remember, when the pants fit comfortably, or loosen, advance with grain reintroduction. If they become tighter, return to a more rigid grain restriction.

For example, Stephanie was able to maintain her weight loss Monday, Tuesday, and Wednesday morning. But when she pulled on her Capris on Thursday morning, they felt a bit snugger than usual. Stephanie went back to the Tuesday quota and followed that indefinitely. Had she continued with the Wednesday levels, she would have continued to gain weight incrementally. Once she increased her level of exercise, she was able to resume adding foods.

On the other hand, Rob was able to eat all the foods through Friday and still maintain his weight loss. For others, it will never be safe to eat grains. Even though some do contain excellent nutrients, due to a combination of genetics and the damage done to your system by years of grain and sugar assault, *your* body may not be able to cope with them without going into an insulin tailspin. Yes, in principle, they are healthy. Other nutritionists or doctors may advise that people eat them. But *your* body can't handle them and they are not healthy for *you*. Fortunately, after going through the first two phases of this diet, you will have learned that you can live and feel better without them.

As I mentioned earlier, some people require regulated amounts of healthy grains and starches for weight loss. Those people who have taken the Metabolic Profile Quiz (page 79) and moved forward more rapidly into Sustain should follow these same guidelines. The only difference is that if you're eating regulated amounts of grains, starches, and fruits to achieve your weight loss, you'll have to identify the level of consumption at which you can lose weight. Those of you who've already achieved your weight loss goals in Stabilize will be reintroducing carbs at a level where you can *sustain* your weight loss.

For everyone, the key is to gradually reintroduce regulated amounts of, first, starchy vegetables, second, healthy grains, and third, selected fruits—*while weighing yourself daily.* This will help you determine the *exact* level you can eat to feel your best and lose weight (or maintain your weight loss). Follow the chart below to gradually introduce the regulated amounts of, first, allowed starches, next, grains, and finally, fruit in a safe day-by-day fashion. Remember to monitor your weight as well as your mood, cravings, and energy level, in order to determine the ideal quota level for you. If you begin to gain weight, or experience any of the symptoms mentioned above, go back to the previous day and remain there for ongoing weight loss (or weight-loss maintenance).

Carb Quota Monitor			
	STARCHY VEGETABLE, such as yams, squash, carrots, peas, parsnips, beets	HEALTHY GRAINS, such as quinoa, amaranth, millet, oats, teff, buckwheat	APPROVED FRUIT, such as apples, pears, blueberries, grapefruit, lemons, cranberries
MONDAY			
LUNCH	1 TBS		
TUESDAY			
LUNCH	2 TBS		
DINNER	2 TBS		
WEDNESDAY			
BREAKFAST		1 TBS	
LUNCH	3 TBS		
DINNER	1 TBS	1 TBS	
THURSDAY			
BREAKFAST		2 TBS	
LUNCH		½ cup	
DINNER	½ cup		
FRIDAY			
BREAKFAST			one fruit
LUNCH		½ cup	
DINNER		½ cup	

Once you have made this transition, obviously, depending upon your level of activity, you can upgrade your intake of healthy starchy vegetables, grains, and fruits to match your energy output. If, like one patient, you start running marathons, more grains, starches, and fruits will be acceptable—once you have reset your metabolic cycle.

It's Great to Be in Sustain!

If you secretly await Sustain, intending to sneak pancakes, potato chips, cotton candy, or other grain and sugar favorites back into your diet, after a few weeks on the *No-Grain Diet* you may find that these cravings have departed. As your body becomes better nourished, you will progressively lose interest in all of those foods. A year from now, if you happen to sample a former favorite, you may be shocked to discover that it no longer tastes good. Don't be surprised if you never again want to eat starches, sweets, and grains!

Here's why this happens: eating grains and sugars creates a cycle where you want more and more. Replacing them with healthy food *reverses that cycle.* On the *No-Grain Diet,* you use food and EFT to permanently rewire your nervous system circuitry. As a result, your taste buds, instead of leading you astray as they now do, will favor the healthy foods that you need to function optimally.

In Stabilize, you will have attained your ideal weight, with grain cravings banished. However, if you find a new round of temptation surfacing in Sustain, don't be surprised. This can happen if past diets have programmed you to rebound once you relax your vigilance. Eating an omelette at brunch, you may find yourself eyeing your neighbor's waffles. If this happens, don't worry. It doesn't mean your diet has failed. Hidden cravings that resurface can be addressed and eliminated right now. At this critical moment, the Food Plan and EFT can help you get back on track for long-term maintenance. Plus, you can always feel free to reassess your personal fuel mix, as it may change over time.

By now, EFT should be like a trusted friend. Anytime you experience a craving, or face a challenging life situation where you anticipate temptation to eat the wrong foods, turn to your notebook and the EFT chapter, and begin to tap away the feelings that prompt you to eat foods that aren't good for you.

Suppose that a combination of stresses and temptations prompts a major relapse. If this happens, first recognize it. Next, tap away your self-blame with EFT, and third, go back to Start-Up. Begin by setting your weight-loss and health goals, and then head into Start-Up again. The sooner you admit what's happened, the less weight you'll have to lose this time around. Healthy eating is for life, and so is the *No-Grain Diet!*

CHAPTER 6

CUSTOMIZING YOUR DIET (PICK YOUR FOOD PLAN)

In this chapter, I'll show you how to customize the Food Plan to your own needs. I've developed and refined the Food Plan over the last ten years, using it with thousands of people. One thing I've seen is that the *No-Grain Diet* produces spectacular results for the people who try it. But some people are afraid to try it. When I analyzed what was holding them back, I realized that going off grains, while simultaneously eliminating other food supports, was too difficult. Some people needed to move into the diet more gradually. That's why I developed the Booster Food Plan, to help people who met certain health criteria ease more gently into the program.

The Booster Food Plan takes you from where you are to where you want to go. Where you are might be anywhere from slightly over your ideal weight to one hundred pounds or more over it. If where you want to go is toward craving-free slimness and health, the Booster Plan is the place to start—especially if you're concerned about whether or not you can do the Diet. After you've overcome grain addiction, beat cravings, and launched your weight loss, you can move up to the Core and Advanced Food Plans to totally revamp your health. So boost your way up to ultimate weight loss via the Booster Food Plan!

The Booster, Core, and Advanced Food Plans

Here's a brief overview of what the three Food Plans have in common and where they differ.

On all three plans, you will:

• Eliminate grains, starchy foods, and sugars from your diet
• Increase vegetables
• Upgrade consumption of raw vegetables, salads, and juices
• Transition into organic foods
• Eat high-quality proteins
• Eliminate alcohol, artificial sweeteners, and trans-fats
• Transition from coffee to high-quality waters and herbal teas
• Increase consumption of healthy fats and oil supplements

The Booster Food Plan will include:
• An expanded list of transitional protein sources, including selective consumption of dairy products, seafood, soy foods like tofu, and pork products
• Limited consumption of selected fruits and selected starchy vegetables
• Delayed cessation of coffee

The Core Food Plan will move forward into:
• Increased consumption of organic, raw produce
• Vegetable juicing
• Upgrading protein sources to organic
• Eliminating pork products
• Restricting dairy, soy, and seafood selections
• Upgrading supplementation and exercise
• Eliminating fruit (except in Sustain)

The Advanced Food Plan will feature:
• Optimized consumption of organic, raw produce, and juices
• Eliminating shellfish and most commercial dairy
• Coffee and smoking cessation
• Optimized supplementation and exercise
• Expanded health support recommendations

In this next section of this chapter, I'll help you make the final determination about which Food Plan is right for you. It doesn't matter where you start, as long as you *do* start the *No-Grain Diet*. You'll see how easy it is, once you meet real-life people from my patient files who have used the different plans at different times to navigate through various health and dietary concerns and lose all the weight they want.

Your Personal Food Plan

Frankly, I'm an idealist, who would like to better your health and the health of every American—through one of the most powerful tools available to us: food. The *No-Grain Diet* shows you how to do that. As a physician, I would like to see everyone follow the Core Food Plan, while beginning to implement some of my Advanced recommendations. But one thing I've learned is that I can offer my best, but nature, God, the divine, your inner self, whatever you'd like to call it, is in charge of the timing. That's why I created the option for you to easily transition into the diet with the Booster Food Plan, which will allow you to first go *No-Grain* while eating a wider list of food choices, such as dairy products, shellfish, and luncheon meats. On the optimally health-building Core and Advanced Food Plans, you'll attain greater weight loss and lasting health.

Everyone on the *No-Grain Diet* can eat all the foods listed in the Core Food Plan (detailed in the next chapter). If you're ready to begin there, please skip this section and move on to it now. However, depending on your weight-loss goals and your health condition, you can also read on to learn whether the Booster Food Plan or Advanced Food Plan is right for you. The Booster Food Plan is suitable for those in good health seeking modest weight loss. It includes all the items in the Core Food Plan, plus additional options detailed more fully later. For people on the go, beginning with this expanded range of food selections makes it more manageable to incorporate the *No-Grain Diet* principles into one's daily life. The Booster Food Plan gives you the boost you need to launch the *No-Grain Diet*.

On the other hand, those who seek greater weight loss and who suffer from more serious health issues should follow the Advanced Food

Plan, which offers the fastest road to health by eliminating certain foods and upgrading health efforts, which will be further detailed in later chapters of this book. These Advanced options can intensively turn around weight and health issues. Or if you are like me, ready to do whatever it takes to build optimal health, you can achieve it by following the Advanced Food Plan.

Mark was a thirty-nine-year-old photo-stylist with asthma, worsened by an allergy to his cats. Struggling with low energy and chronic depression, he'd seen therapists for nearly a decade and was on antidepressants. Committed to his health, Mark decided to start the Advanced Food Plan. He noticed profound and immediate improvements. After only two weeks, his energy level improved and he started to run regularly, as he had in high school. At his two-month follow-up, Mark weaned himself off of his antidepressant medication. His cat allergy remarkably improved and he only noticed the need for an inhaler once or twice a week—usually when he went off the eating plan. Overall Mark was thrilled, and told me that he felt like he could live to be a hundred.

While some people, like Mark, have a level of commitment and a lifestyle that supports healthy changes, for others change needs to be more gradual—and that's just fine. What's important is to recognize where you are, and begin *there*. You are the best judge of what works for you.

Which Is the Right Food Plan for Me?

Perhaps life stresses make it hard for you to implement more than a few changes at once. Maybe you doubt your ability to do the Advanced Food Plan, and need to build confidence or address doubts. Whatever the case, if you'd like to begin with the Booster Food Plan, I want you to do it safely and successfully. That's why I've developed some criteria for making that choice.

It is safe to undertake the Booster Food Plan depending on these four factors:

1. Your Goals Assessment questionnaire results (see page 93)
2. The size of your weight gain
3. Your health condition
4. Lab tests, if needed (see recommended tests in Chapter Five)

I created a Goals Assessment questionnaire, included later in this chapter, to help you see where you are. By filling it out, you'll be able to more specifically determine what's appropriate for you. But briefly, here's an overview of what to consider for each Food Plan.

The Booster Food Plan, described more fully in this and the next chapter, is appropriate if:

- You are in good health.
- Your weight-loss goals are relatively modest (twenty pounds or less).
- Your weight gain is not long-standing (two years or less).
- You are not diabetic.
- You do not have a serious health condition requiring more immediate treatment.

The Core Food Plan is the way to go if:

- You feel highly dedicated to your weight and health goals.
- Your weight loss goals are more ambitious.
- Your weight gain over and above your target weight is long-standing. (You've weighed twenty pounds or more above your target weight for over two years.)
- You have any health issues.
- You are diabetic.
- You have high blood pressure or heart disease.
- You have irritable bowel syndrome or other chronic digestive disorders.
- You have allergies.

The Advanced Food Plan is for you if:

- You are ready to commit to optimal health.
- You have long-standing weight gain (five years or more).
- You are overweight by more than fifty pounds.
- You have any autoimmune condition. (See box.)
- You have any chronic degenerative health problem that hasn't been helped by a conventional medical approach.
- You have any of the following more serious health conditions:
  —Most cancers
  —Heart disease
  —Fibromyalgia
  —Chronic fatigue syndrome
  —Chronic infections, including yeast problems and potentially life-threatening infections like hepatitis C
  —Any of the autoimmune diseases mentioned in the chart below

---

Autoimmune Diseases Listed by the Main Target Organ

Nervous System
Multiple sclerosis
Myasthenia gravis
Guillain-Barré
Autoimmune uveitis

Blood
Autoimmune
   hemolytic anemia
Pernicious anemia

Blood Vessels
Temporal arteritis
Anti-phospholipid
   syndrome
Wegener's
   granulomatosis
Behcet's disease

Gastrointestinal System
Crohn's disease
Ulcerative colitis
Primary biliary cirrhosis
Autoimmune hepatitis

**Multiple Organs and
Musculoskeletal System**
Rheumatoid arthritis
Systemic lupus
   erythematosus
Scleroderma
Polymyositis
   Dermatomyositis
Ankylosing spondylitis
Sjogren's syndrome

Endocrine Glands
Type 1 or immune-mediated
   diabetes mellitus
Grave's disease
Hashimoto's thyroiditis
Autoimmune oophoritis and
   orchitis
Autoimmune adrenal
   disease

Skin
Psoriasis
Dermatitis herpetiformis
Pemphigus vulgaris
Vitiligo

In addition to undergoing the Goals Assessment, I encourage you to consult your doctor or health care professional for further guidance, and to take the lab tests I discussed in Chapter Five. These can really home in on your current state of health.

Goals Assessment				
Your Intention (Circle One)	A	B	C	D
1. How motivated are you?				
A. I'm somewhat motivated	2			
B. I'm very motivated		10		
C. I'm totally determined			25	
Your Weight Loss				
2. How many pounds overweight are you?				
A. 10–15 pounds	2			
B. 15–50 pounds		10		
C. 50 pounds +			20	
3. How long have you been overweight?				
A. Under two years	2			
B. Over two years		10		
C. Since the age of sixteen or under			20	
4. What is your target weight-loss goal?				
A. 10–15 pounds	2			
B. 15–50 pounds		10		
C. 50 pounds +			25	
5. If you answered B or C, how soon do you intend to reach your target weight?				
A. Eventually	2			
B. As soon as possible		25		
Grain Addiction				
6. How many servings of grains, starches, and sweets do you eat each day?				
A. Two servings or less	5			
B. Three to five servings		10		
C. More than five servings			15	

(continued)

Grain Addiction (*continued*)	A	B	C	D
7. I use grains, starches, or sweets to calm, comfort, or nurture myself.				
A. Never to rarely	5			
B. Sometimes		10		
C. Regularly			20	
8. I've been on the *No-Grain Diet.*				
A. Never	5			
B. For over three months successfully		10		
C. Tried Start-Up but can't stay on it			20	
Health Condition				
9. My health is:				
A. Excellent	30			
B. Average to good with noticeable complaints		0		
C. Fair; I have some minor problems			10	
D. I have a serious health issue				25
10. Please add thirty points each if you have been diagnosed with any of the following illnesses:				
• Autoimmune disorders, including rheumatoid arthritis, inflammatory bowel disease, and others				
• Neurological disorders, such as Parkinson's, Alzheimer's, or MS				
• Any chronic degenerative health problem				
11. Please add fifty points each if you have been diagnosed with any of the following illnesses:				
• Cancer				
• Heart or other cardiovascular disease				
• Type 2 diabetes				
12. Family History: Please add five points for each immediate family member (parent, grandparent, or sibling) who has suffered from any of the above-mentioned illnesses.				

(*continued*)

Scores:
Add up your scores.
If you have scored 30–50 points, you can safely start with the
Booster Food Plan.
If you have 50–90 points, you should do the Core Food Plan.
If you have 90 points or more, proceed to the Advanced Food Plan.

As long as you score below 50 points on the questionnaire and meet the criteria mentioned below, you can use the Booster Food Plan. If you scored between 50 and 90 points, you should begin with the Core Food Plan. And if you scored above 90 points, you should go with the Advanced Food Plan.

In addition, if you scored in the Advanced range, or if you have any of the illnesses or risk factors indicated above in the Health Condition portion of the questionnaire (or in the preceding guidelines), I strongly advise you to take the medical tests for blood pressure, cholesterol, thyroid, and insulin levels. You should take them before starting the diet to establish a baseline, and then as often as every eight weeks during Stabilize. Once your tests results have stabilized at desirable levels, you are ready to wait four weeks and then move on to Sustain.

Monitoring yourself emotionally and physically is central to the *No-Grain Diet*. Obviously, I would like you to undertake the most advanced level comfortable for you. At the same time, whichever level you choose, you'll receive the major benefits of this program. Whenever your goals change, you can reevaluate and either accelerate or de-accelerate your program.

So, Doctor, What Do You Recommend?

All variations of the diet guarantee you weight loss, renewed energy, and improved health. The difference is in degree. If you've ever used a treadmill at the gym, you know that you can adapt your workout by adjusting your speed and incline. You build strength more slowly by going at a more relaxed pace. Or you can build at a more accelerated pace, with a steeper curve that delivers more powerful results. The choice is yours. And it's just the same on the *No-Grain Diet*.

The modifications allow you to work the plan at your own speed and your own rate. The Advanced Food Plan puts you into high-gear health, and can also help give your body the optimized nutrition necessary to reverse many serious health conditions.

If you have any kind of serious health condition, I advise you to take the plunge into the Advanced Food Plan. If you feel you need to, you can spend a few weeks on the Core Food Plan to acclimate yourself, but for solid results you should move into the more accelerated program as soon as possible.

Michele was a thirty-three-year-old elementary school teacher whose health problems had prevented her from working for over six years. She weighed 254 pounds and had developed Type 2 diabetes. She was on medication for depression, had multiple digestive problems, and irregular periods. Michele had been diagnosed with fibromyalgia, chronic fatigue immune dysfunction (CFIDS), and Hashimoto's thyroiditis.

We both agreed that she had serious health problems and should aim for the Advanced Food Plan, but she started on the Core Food Plan for one month as she adjusted to having four ounces of juice in the morning. One month after starting the *No-Grain Diet*, which she followed completely, Michele had lost twelve pounds and normalized her blood sugar levels, so that she was able to go off her diabetic medication. After two months, she had lost an additional fifteen pounds and discontinued her antidepressants. With renewed energy, she was able to return to her job. She now has a life and feels very grateful. She continues to use EFT both for the occasional craving and to reengineer her self-image to that of a healthy woman who can enjoy life.

As you can see from Michele's story, the *No-Grain Diet* is very powerful, so powerful that it can turn around a major weight gain along with reversing a combination of serious illnesses, as it did in Michele's case. Just imagine that powerful health engine at work in your life!

On the other hand, you may be in good health and only slightly over your target weight. You have many demands in your life, and for you, it's easier to go *No-Grain* while having the flexibility to enjoy a shrimp cocktail at a professional conference or eat a bit more cheese than would be strictly optimal. You'd like to be able to make vegetable juice, but right now it's more practical to make a protein drink or grab a yogurt. The Booster Food Plan contains all those options.

Once past grain elimination on the Booster Food Plan, you can work your way into the Core Food Plan, by cutting back on the expanded Booster Food options when you are ready. Once you've addressed your grain addiction, launched your weight loss, and become confident in using EFT, you'll find it easier to take the time you need to move up and on to ever more optimal Food Plans. In the next chapter, I'll explain why some of the foods you'll still enjoy on the Booster Plan have unexpected downsides; you may choose to reduce and eliminate them over time. But your chief priority will be to overcome your addictions and put grains, starches, and sweets behind you.

Let's take a look at how this could work. Suppose you've started with the Booster Food Plan and gotten good results; after a few weeks (or more) you may want to consider advancing your program and moving up to the Core Food Plan. Ask yourself if you're ready and listen quietly to what your body tells you. If you feel at peace, with no anxiety or distress, you're ready to move ahead. If not, you might turn to EFT to address the emotions and concerns that block you from moving forward. When you're ready, I encourage you to consider upgrading the program to maximize your health benefits and feel better than you ever have before.

Olivia was a thirty-nine-year old woman who felt tired and couldn't lose the twenty-five pounds she'd gained after her son's birth seven years earlier. Although other doctors told her that her thyroid was normal, the more sophisticated thyroid tests I do in my practice revealed that it was functioning below par.

When she started the *No-Grain Diet,* at first Olivia experienced chocolate cravings, but EFT helped her to overcome her sugar addiction. She soon noticed her cravings for bagels and pizza had also disappeared, and she lost seven pounds her first month on the Diet. Feeling full of energy, Olivia was ready to move up to the Core Food Plan. After seven months, she reached her ideal body weight and told me, "I feel like I did in high school!"

Upgrading her exercise, Olivia began to run in local 5K races, and when we last met, she was a model of health, who now influences her family and friends to consider making changes in their own eating habits.

How to Move Between Food Plans

This is a diet you will follow for a lifetime, so as things in your life change, so should your diet. I don't want you to view this plan as a rigid dictum. I want you to make the Diet your own, and to know how to respond to whatever needs arise.

Now, let's suppose that you've been on the Core Food Plan and made some solid gains. Recently, due to life stresses, you've lapsed from the diet. Instead of beating yourself up, which makes restarting even more of a challenge, give yourself a fresh start by going back to Start-Up with your choice of either the Booster or Core Food Plan. Returning to Start-Up will ease you back into the *No-Grain Diet* in a supported way. And don't forget to use EFT so that you immediately stop blaming yourself for your lapse!

While it's easy to bounce back once the stress is over, let's face reality. Sometimes stress seems to hang around a long time. Whether it's job pressures, family concerns, relationship problems, unexpected health issues, or financial worries, at one time or another most of us find ourselves in an ongoing stress state for months or even years. When that happens, it's easy to begin a backslide, turning to comfort foods to help us through tough times.

If at any point you realize that, provoked by stress, you've returned to old patterns, let me reassure you that you haven't blown the diet. In fact, congratulations for recognizing it, since that's the first step back to health.

When Irene came to see me, tests showed that she had a blood glucose level of 119, veering dangerously close to diabetic levels. Moreover, with a family history of diabetes, Irene couldn't afford to continue eating the way she had: grabbing a Danish and coffee for breakfast, more coffee with a lunchtime sandwich. Because of her busy work schedule, dinner was often frozen pizza or pasta popped into the microwave. After a few weeks on the Booster Food Plan, Irene successfully transitioned into the Core Food Plan, and maintained it for over a year. Enjoying a protein drink for breakfast, a healthy salad with chicken, turkey, or a burger for lunch, and an array of healthy protein and vegetable dinners, Irene had slimmed down and was enjoying renewed energy in her life.

All was going well, until the head of her company resigned, triggering a company-wide reorganization that threatened many jobs. As an HR person, Irene was under siege, working late hours, addressing a lot of fear and emotional pain. Not surprisingly, under these demands, Irene began to creep off the Diet. First, it was an afternoon coffee, then it was a cookie to go with it. Soon the hurried luncheon sandwich replaced her healthy salad. As Irene's energy dipped, she naturally began to drink more coffee.

Irene felt guilty about blowing the diet, but her guilt wasn't helping her get back on board; it was keeping her off the diet, as she spiraled into self-blame, and ate to make herself feel better. When I pointed this out, Irene admitted her feelings, and began the first step: she used EFT to help overcome them. Once the guilt and tension had subsided, Irene felt better about herself. Recognizing that drinking coffee to bolster her sagging energy was key, Irene began daily use of EFT to address her on-the-job stress, performing it before her workday and during five-minute breaks. As a result she felt more energized and more in control. She decided to go back to Start-Up using the Booster Food Plan. By cutting herself some slack, she transitioned easily back into the program, and soon was managing her job stresses while moving into the Core Food Plan. She added regular exercise, and gained strength and confidence as she held her own in a stressed environment. Irene's can-do attitude was a standout in her company, and an encounter with a recruiter opened the door to a higher-level job in a better-managed firm.

As you can see in Irene's situation, the *No-Grain Diet* can support you through life's challenges. The key is flexibility, and turning to the program tools whenever you need them.

In the next chapter, you'll be learning the most powerful tool of all: the Diet itself. You'll find out just what foods to eat—and to avoid—on the Booster, Core, and Advanced Food Plans. With this knowledge, you'll achieve weight-loss goals, rebuild your health, and maximize your energy.

CHAPTER 7

THE FOOD PLAN (ALL THE FOODS YOU CAN EAT)

You've learned the basic structure of the Diet; let's focus more closely on what you'll actually be eating. The recipes and menu plans (which you'll find in Parts 2 and 4 of this book) make the diet easy and enjoyable. They are designed to nourish you, eliminate hunger, and reprogram your cells. Your meals and snacks will assure that never again will bodily cells screaming for fuel prompt you to reach for the wrong food. You'll be better nourished than ever before, with more energy for the tasks of life. What's more, on this diet, you'll build confidence and positive self-esteem as you gain control of your weight loss.

As you learned in the previous chapters, during Start-Up you eat every two hours, and during Stabilize you eat five to six meals a day. Frequent meals stop your hunger. In this chapter, I'll familiarize you with the foods you can and cannot eat, while providing you with important tips for incorporating this new way of eating into your life.

Next, I'll introduce you to the basic food groups that make up the Booster, Core, and Advanced Food Plans. You will be eating *all of the foods* detailed on these lists, and avoiding foods and food types not on them. At first, you'll go through a process of adjusting to the restrictions, and I advise you to use EFT as a support. But soon you'll get accustomed to your food list. You'll be eating large quantities of the allowed vegetables and incorporating more raw vegetables into your diet. In addition, you'll be exercising and using some of the supplements

I recommend in the next chapter. After a few weeks, you'll find tremendous freedom as the *No-Grain Diet* works for you. This Diet is simple and easy to follow. Counting calories or carbohydrate grams is not a requirement because the foods are so filling and satisfying that it will be very hard for you to eat a large enough quantity of, say, broccoli to gain weight. All the work is done for you.

Why Organic?

Ideally half of your produce, protein, and fats should be organic. Don't be misled by media reports questioning the value of organic foods. The simple facts are: Synthetic fertilizers have depleted nutrients in our farmland such that *ordinary produce lacks vitamins and minerals.* Pesticides used in mass agribusiness kill bugs because they are *poisons.* Now FDA studies confirm that our nonorganic food is contaminated with these very same pesticides/poisons. You can avoid them by consuming organic foods because they:

- Contain less pesticides than nonorganic produce
- Contain significantly higher levels of vitamins and minerals
- Help revitalize the land
- Support family farmers
- Taste delicious!

In deciding what you'll eat, you affect not only your personal health, but also the health of the planet. Conventional agriculture is a major source of the environmental pollution that corrupts our streams, rivers, and lakes. To have a cleaner and healthier body, you need a cleaner and healthier environment. If we pollute the air, water, and land, ultimately we pollute ourselves. Choosing organic foods is one small step toward a healthier life and world. If its too costly for you, begin gradually. Once you taste the difference, you might find surprising ways to stay on the organic track!

Eat More Vegetables

Protein diets have been around for years, but this one is different because of its strong accent on vegetables. Not all carbohydrates are created equal. It's a mistake to focus solely on carbohydrate content as the measurement of a food, without taking into account the type of carbohydrate and the effect it produces in the body.

In avoiding grains that rapidly turn to sugar in the body, we can stabilize the insulin cycle. But we lose out on vital nutrients when we shun complex carb foods that don't trigger that insulin reaction. To prevent a sunburn, you should avoid sitting outdoors in the sunlight at high noon in August. But does that mean you should stay indoors, recoiling from daylight at all times?

Of course not. Similarly, on this diet, you'll eat generous quantities of vegetables because they promote health. It's far more beneficial to increase your vegetable intake than to take vitamins. Vegetables contain phytochemicals, powerful natural agents used by the body to cleanse, repair, and build healthy cells, organs, and tissues. They contain fiber, which gives a feeling of fullness after a meal and cleanses your digestion. You can optimize your body's pH acid/alkaline balance by eating approximately one pound of vegetables every day for every 100 pounds of body weight. That means: if you weigh 150 pounds, eat one and one half pounds of vegetables. However, you can fine-tune further, by eating more or less than this quantity, guided by your own appetite and comfort level. Remember that this is a general guideline, based on the average person. You can experiment to discover what's right for you. Once again, organic produce is healthiest, so each successive Food Plan upgrades your intake of organic vegetables.

Because cooking and processing can destroy essential food micronutrients by altering their shape and chemical composition, I want you to also increase the amount of raw vegetables you eat. Monitor your body's reaction to assure that they agree with you, and if not, start by lightly steaming them. Eventually, you will become accustomed to eating more substantial amounts. Fresh squeezed juices, raw salads, and blended soups are excellent ways to incorporate raw foods into your diet. You'll find instructions and recipes later in this book. Nearly all vegetables can be eaten raw, including broccoli, cauliflower, and others we typically cook. But feel free to begin with familiar raw food favorites, like cucumbers, spinach, and avocado.

Raw Juices and Vegetables

Begin with 20 percent of your daily vegetables eaten raw, and then gradually increase to 50 percent. Steadily increasing your consumption of vegetable juice is one of the best ways to boost your vegetable intake to desirable levels.

Freshly processed vegetable juices have multiple benefits. They:

Alkalinize and rebalance your body's pH
Increase your energy level
Help improve your immune system
Heal and prevent chronic diseases

For complete instructions on juicing, including my recommendations on the best kinds of juicers to purchase, see the Resources section. For juicing recipes, see Part 4.

If you have trouble digesting vegetables, or experience gas, constipation, or other digestive discomfort, begin slowly and build up to the desired amount. If you are allergic to specific vegetables, eliminate them from your diet for at least three months. Later, you may find that you have rebuilt your immune system strength and no longer need to avoid them.

In general, the greener the vegetable, the better. Green vegetables are filled with chlorophyll, the plant storage system for sunshine. Emphasize leafy greens like Swiss chard, collard greens, and bok choy. Watery, white iceberg lettuce has little nutritional value and isn't worth the time it takes to chew.

Is every vegetable good? No. High-starch vegetables, like potatoes, or their products, including fries and potato chips, function just like grains, turning rapidly to glucose in your body. They are not allowed on this diet.

What about carrots and beets, the prime ingredients in that old health-food-store standby, carrot juice? Sweet root vegetables like these function as "turncoats." Their sweetness quickly turns to glucose in the body, triggering an undesirable insulin spike. On the Booster Food Plan, you are allowed to eat a minimal serving of carrots, such as the amount in a cup of vegetable soup or minestrone. Carrots are more harmful in their juiced form, because of the larger concentration of blood sugar stimulation than you'd get from eating a single carrot. For the Core and Advanced Food Plans, please avoid them until Sustain, when they can be selectively reintroduced by those who are stable in their weight and health goals.

Approved Vegetables to Eat Often on All Food Plans
Asparagus, kale, kohlrabi, Swiss chard, collards, spinach, dandelion greens, green and red cabbage, broccoli, red and green leaf lettuce, romaine lettuce, endive, escarole, parsley, radishes, broccoli rabe, radicchio, scallions, Chinese cabbage, bok choy, fennel, celery, cucumbers, cauliflower, zucchini, Brussels sprouts, tomatoes, turnips, and green, yellow, and red peppers

Vegetables to Avoid
Iceberg lettuce
Carrots
Potatoes and beets, squashes
Corn (really a grain)

Replace Grains with Vegetables

On the Start-Up and Stabilize phases of this diet, you eliminate all grains, including wheat, rice, millet, spelt, oats, quinoa, teff, and amaranth, and their products. You will also eliminate every food prepared from them, such as corn products, like popcorn, tacos, or chips, as well as *everything made with flour:* bread, pasta, pizza, crackers, pancakes, cakes, rice cakes, cookies, pies—in short, the whole enchilada.

As you now realize, for anyone who weighs more than they should, grains and starches are harmful and unnecessary. However, for under-weight people, or people far into the Sustain part of the Diet, whole grains like those mentioned above can promote health. However, their flour-based offspring are still undesirable.

Fruits

Once you are in the Sustain phase of the Diet, the following fruits are permitted, but no more than one piece of fruit per day. Fruits are cleansing and contain vital antioxidants; however, it's important to limit consumption because of the natural sugars within them. It's best to eat small pieces throughout the day to prevent a rapid rise in blood sugar. Fruit is not allowed in Start-Up and Stabilize, except on the Booster Food Plan, when you may consume up to three pieces of fruit per week chosen from the limited Booster fruits. Fruit juice is never permitted because of the excessive amount of sugar.

Booster Food Plan

**Approved Fruits for Start-Up and Stabilize
(Eat no more than three fruits per week)**

Granny Smith apple	Lemon
Cranberry	Lime
Grapefruit	

Booster, Core, and Modified Food Plans

**Approved *No-Grain Diet* Fruit Chart
for Sustain Only**

Apple	Melons (Cantaloupe)
Apricot	Mulberries
Avocado	Nectarine
Banana	Olives
Blueberries	Orange
Cherries	Papaya
Cranberries	Peach
Grapefruit	Pear

(continued)

**Approved *No-Grain Diet* Fruit Chart
for Sustain Only *(continued)***

Grapes	Pineapple
Kiwi	Plum
Lemon	Raspberries
Lime	Strawberries
Mango	Watermelon

Proteins

In addition to a strong component of healthful vegetables, the *No-Grain Diet* emphasizes protein. Your protein needs vary according to your sex, height, weight, and exercise levels, with increased consumption beneficial for most people. Normal ranges are from twenty grams (a three-ounce serving of most meats) to fifty grams (a seven-ounce serving) at each meal. A one-hundred-pound woman under five feet tall will need twenty grams daily, while a three-hundred-pound six-foot-six-inch football player would require closer to fifty grams per meal. But once again, you will determine your requirements based on your personal fuel mix.

However, it's important not to *overeat* protein, as excess protein can weaken kidney function and decrease bone density. As protein is digested, it turns to acid in the body; minerals are leeched from the bones to compensate. However, the quantities of vegetables you'll consume on this diet prevent bone demineralization. What's more, you can always supplement with calcium and magnesium to maintain bone mass.

The Healthiest Proteins

Eggs

An excellent source of protein, eggs are recommended on all three Food Plans. Organic eggs are best since they contain a 1:1 omega 6 to 3 ratio, while commercial eggs contain a 20:1 omega 6 to 3 ratio. It's the excessive omega 6 fats, not the cholesterol, that make commercial eggs unhealthy. While organic eggs are preferred, you can still eat commercial eggs, if necessary, but consume them less frequently. Your cooking method determines whether you absorb oxidized cholesterol, a precursor to clogged arteries and heart disease, or not. *High heating promotes oxidation,* which also occurs when the iron in the egg white combines with the egg yolk. That's why scrambled eggs and omelets should be eaten only rarely. However, if you keep your yolks intact and cook eggs over low heat, you'll avoid that problem. Cook them only until the yolks are runny, as in soft boiling, poaching, or sunny side up. Do not eat them more than five out of seven days, to avoid developing an allergy. If you are doing the Advanced Food Plan for optimal health, you can begin to incorporate raw egg yolks into your juice. Please check the Resources section (and my website) for instructions on how to do that safely.

Organic Meat

In recent years, bacterial strains resistant to all but a few antibiotics are increasingly common, due to worldwide *overuse* of antibiotics, experts believe. The result: ever more virulent bugs fight off the antibiotics we use to check them. Conventionally raised cattle are fed antibiotics, increasing resistance in *humans* through the transfer of antibiotic-resistant bacteria in meat. In addition, it's common to feed hormones to our poultry and livestock.

I recommend that you consume only grass-fed beef, along with organic poultry and meat. Organic poultry, lamb, and beef can be found in many health food stores, as well as on the Internet.

Meat Choices

Buffalo/bison, venison, and lamb are good options since they are game animals and have fewer pesticides. Ostrich, chicken, and turkey are also good protein sources.

Grass-Fed Beef

While eating *grain-fed* beef is better than grain consumption, authentic *grass-fed* beef is a far superior protein source. Why is feeding cattle *grass* so important? A cow's traditional diet *is* grass, which is high in the beneficial omega-3 fats. Eating grass-fed beef gives you both protein and omega-3 fats, a vital dietary component I'll explain further when I discuss fats in this and the next chapter. Corn, the current staple of commercially raised cows, is high in omega-6 fats, which create an unfavorable ratio of healthy to non-optimal fats, for both the animals and *you* (if you eat them). As I'll discuss more fully, normalizing your omega 6:3 ratio is one of the keys to improving your health. What's more, cattle in commercial feedlots are fed corn to fatten them up. Guess what: if you eat that meat, it will fatten *you* up.

That's why I suggest you consume meat raised on natural grasses. However, it's hard to find, and often "so-called" grass-fed beef is not. Unless you can check with a cattle farmer whom you know and trust, you may not get the real thing, which is why I took the trouble to identify authentic sources and offer real grass-fed beef on my website.

Protein Powders

Although useful for those on the run, protein powders are highly processed and do not provide the full benefits of real food. If you use them, avoid soy protein (for reasons I'll clarify), and instead use a high-quality whey or rice protein. Study the ingredients carefully, as fructose or other sugars are often added.

Whey proteins, derived from milk, are an excellent protein source, without the usual allergies provoked by dairy, since they lack casein. Most people who don't tolerate milk do fine with the whey protein powder.

Rice protein, a predigested protein source, is also excellent and, surprisingly, contains pure protein, with no harmful carbohydrates to raise insulin levels. Remember, grains themselves are not intrinsically evil. Consult the appendix for additional protein powders I recommend to my patients.

Healthy Protein Sources

Whey Protein
　Bio Pure Whey Protein from Metagenics
Rice Protein
　Nutrabiotic Rice Protein

(continued)

Healthy Protein Sources (*continued*)

Yeast
Consisting of 50 percent protein and loaded with natural B vitamins, yeast powders are relatively inexpensive.
- Twin Labs Genuine Brewer's Yeast Powder
- Vegetrates Brewer's Yeast Flakes
- Lewis Labs Brewer's Yeast Powder

Spirulina
Spirulina is a microalgae, consisting of 60 percent protein.
- Powder Earthrise Certified Spirulina
- Nutrex Hawaiian Spirulina Powder

Healthy Proteins? Not!

Certain standard protein sources, commonly highlighted in other "healthy diets," such as dairy, seafood, soy products, and nuts, I consider less than optimal. This surprises many people who undertake the Diet, because they've been told that these are "health foods." Although they have some health benefits, they have some significant downsides, which I'll explain further. Please note that the Booster Food Plan is more permissive regarding these foods, and you can eat small amounts of them (at one meal and two snacks per day). As you move into the Core Food Plan, I recommend limiting or eliminating them entirely.

Fish

Up until very recently, I considered fish a staple of a healthy diet. But now, despite its beneficial fats and nutrients, fish are so contaminated with mercury, PCBs, and DDT that I can't wholeheartedly endorse them. Mercury is so toxic that only a few milligrams can kill you. In the U.S. alone, every year industry releases more than 5 million pounds of mercury compounds into the environment. This mercury changes into an even more toxic compound, known as methyl mercury. As fish eat plankton and smaller fish, which have absorbed methyl mercury from contaminated bodies of water, it builds up in their bodies, and gets passed along to you with every fish dinner. Our lack of vigilance in protecting our environment has now traveled directly to the dinner table, where we are forced to limit our intake of this favorite food. Having ordered thousands of hair mineral analyses to detect mercury absorption, I can tell you that nearly all fish are highly contaminated. The only exception I have found to date, is the wild salmon from a company called Vital Choice Seafood.

Obviously, pregnant women and people with serious health conditions should avoid fish completely. In general, don't make fish a staple of your diet, unless you're absolutely certain it has been lab-tested and shown to be free of detectable levels of mercury and other toxins. Make sure to consume only modest amounts of the less contaminated fish recommended here.

Fish to Avoid

Swordfish	Gulf coast oysters
Shark	Marlin
King mackerel	Halibut
Tilefish	Pike
Tuna	Walleye
Sea bass	White croaker

Approved *No-Grain Diet* Fish on All Food Plans

Summer flounder	Sardines
Wild pacific salmon	Haddock
Croaker	Mackerel
Cod	Tilapia

In general, I recommend avoiding shellfish (lobsters, crabs, shrimp, etc.), which are scavengers and frequently contaminated with parasites and viruses. Occasional use on the Booster Food Plan is permitted.

Seeds and Nuts

When you eat seeds and nuts, choose walnuts and flaxseeds. Except for walnuts, almost all nuts contain high levels of omega-6 fats, which, if eaten in excess, can unbalance your body's omega-6 to omega-3 fat ratio. For reasons I'll explain in depth later in this chapter and Chapter

Nine, most of us already have too much omega-6 fat. Unless you are very healthy, it's important to restrict your intake. Walnuts, though permitted, should be used sparingly, to assure weight loss. Several tablespoons of freshly ground flaxseeds added to salads, juices, or soups, can help normalize your digestion, whether you are constipated or have loose bowels. You can also mix them into water, and drink them as you would Metamucil. A wider range of nuts is permitted on the Booster Food Plan, but please use them for rare treats, such as the desserts allowed on Sustain.

Soy

Unless it is fermented or sprouted, soy is *not* a health food. Despite its beneficial properties, it contains digestive enzyme inhibitors that impair your ability to break down protein, as well as phytic acid, which binds minerals and prevents their absorption. Sprouting (of soy sprouts) and fermentation (found in tempeh, natto, and miso) eliminate these harmful factors, and these are excellent protein sources, which is why they are recommended soy foods. (For recipes, see Chapter Twelve.)

Tempeh (available in the dairy or frozen food section at most health food stores) comes in many different flavors. Oven braising (see recipes, Chapter Twelve) moderates its strong taste so that it can be used in burgers, meat loaves, and chilis. Miso, the key ingredient in the popular Japanese miso soup, donates a rich, salty flavor to soups, stews, and vegetable dishes.

Natto, made of fermented soybeans, is sold in Asian or Japanese food markets. Despite its strong smell and egg yolk–like consistency, it has a high concentration of vitamin K, which helps blood clotting, improves bone density, and is commonly used for osteoporosis in Japan.

I don't recommend tofu, soy protein products, and soymilk. If you do eat these products, you should only eat a modest amount, and only if you are on the Booster Food Plan.

Soy Protein Powders

Avoid soy protein and instead use a high-quality whey or rice protein.

Beans and Legumes

Unless you have a high insulin level, you can eat beans, which contain both carbohydrates and proteins. Since beans only have a partial range of amino acids, the building blocks of protein, at the same meal make sure to eat additional proteins. As well, make sure to soak your beans overnight and discard the soak water to remove harmful phytates which make them indigestible. If you have a problem digesting them, you can also easily obtain raw beans (from a health food store) and sprout them. To sprout beans, first soak them overnight, then drain. Next, allow them to sprout in a bowl, jar, or colander, rinsing and draining them three times daily. They will cook more quickly and be easier to digest afterward.

Dairy

Most people benefit from stopping dairy, so avoid dairy for a few weeks to see if your health symptoms improve. If you can tolerate dairy, restrict yourself to goat, sheep, and or raw cow's milk cheese. Raw (unpasteurized) milk is good if you can obtain it from healthy sources. Although small amounts of cheddar, mozzarella, Swiss, and Roquefort, and other blue cheeses are allowed, stop all other commercial milk products, including skim milk and ice cream, as well as rice milk, soymilk, Lactaid, and acidophilus milk.

Although yogurt is allowed, steer clear of low-fat dairy products and sweetened yogurt due to their high carbohydrate content. Unsweetened sheep or goat's milk is preferred. Why don't I encourage use of a supposedly healthy food like yogurt? Yogurt is made from milk, which is pasteurized and homogenized to protect us from E. coli and other bacteria. These procedures change the delicate structure of its proteins and nutrients, making them hard to digest. Many of my patients from India consumed yogurt in their native land with no problem until they immigrated to the U.S. Eating yogurt here, they developed severe digestive problems like IBS (irritable bowel syndrome), which only abated when they stopped eating yogurt.

Approved *No-Grain Diet* Dairy List on All Food Plans

Sheep or goat's milk and cheese

Plain cow organic yogurt

Plain goat's or sheep's milk yogurt

Raw milk cheese

Cheddar or Colby cheese

Feta cheese (sheep or goat derived)

Blue cheese

Skim mozzarella cheese

Whole milk mozzarella cheese

Grated parmesan cheese

Swiss cheese

Skim ricotta

Cream

Milk

Sour cream

Pork

Pigs are scavenger animals, frequently contaminated with parasites that are not removed by cooking. Pork fat often contains mold spores. Avoid all ham and pork products, although limited servings are permitted on the Booster Food Plan.

Approved *No-Grain Diet* Proteins

Booster Food Plan

Grass-fed beef

Ostrich

Poultry: chicken, turkey, duck

Game meats: buffalo (bison), lamb

Pork and luncheon meats, restricted use

Eggs, organic preferred; nonorganic, pasteurized egg whites or egg substitute products acceptable

Dairy: cheeses, raw and goat cheeses preferred; Cheddar, Colby, mozzarella, Parmesan, Swiss, and ricotta, in limited quantities; milk, cream, sour cream, and plain yogurt in limited quantities; avoid low-fat dairy products

Beans and legumes: all

Raw seeds: all, flax preferred

Raw nuts: all, walnuts preferred

Protein powder: all

Soy: all, fermented soy products preferred

Fish: all approved fish; shellfish eaten sparingly

Core Food Plan

Grass-fed beef

Ostrich

Poultry: chicken, turkey, duck

Game meats: buffalo, lamb

Eggs: organic and omega-3 preferred

Dairy: cheeses, raw and goat cheeses preferred; Cheddar, Colby, mozzarella, Parmesan, Swiss, and ricotta, in limited quantities; milk, cream, sour cream, and plain yogurt in limited quantities; avoid low-fat dairy products

Raw seeds: flax

Raw nuts: walnuts

Beans and legumes: lentils, chickpeas, adzuki beans once a week only

Soy: eliminate, except for fermented soy products (miso, tempeh, and soy sprouts)

Protein powder: no soy powders

Fish: all approved fish

Eliminate pork: ham, most bacon, pork roast, and chops

Eliminate shellfish: shrimp, lobster, crabs, clams

Advanced Food Plan

Grass-fed beef

Ostrich

Poultry: chicken, turkey, ostrich

Game meats: buffalo, lamb

Eggs: organic and omega-3 preferred

Dairy: eliminate except for raw sources

Raw seeds: flax

Raw nuts: walnuts

Beans and legumes: eliminate

Eliminate soy, except for fermented soy products (miso, tempeh, and soy sprouts)

Protein powder: whey and rice protein only

Fish: salmon, cod, mackerel, eaten sparingly

Eliminate pork: ham, most bacon, pork roast, and chops

Eliminate shellfish: shrimp, lobster, crabs, clams

Eat the Right Fats

For decades we've heard that fats are the culprits in countless diseases, although no research actually demonstrates the correlation between fatty foods and increased health risk. Yet, at the behest of our medical advisors, we've been cutting out fats, and the net result is increased consumption of fattening and health-damaging starches and sugars.

As I discussed in earlier chapters of this book, a growing body of medical evidence points in the opposite direction, and it's now clear that you must eat the right fats both for your health and to lose weight. Increasing omega-3 fats, found in fatty fish, fish oils, flaxseeds, and grass-fed, free-range livestock and poultry, is essential. Since your brain is about 60 percent fat, the fats you eat strongly enhance brain cell membranes and functioning. Omega-3 fats, DHA and EPA, are essential to brain and nerve function. Some nutritional anthropologists believe the human brain would not have developed as it did without access to the high levels of DHA found in fish and the vital organs of wild game.

For cooking, I recommend coconut oil, which when heated does not become a trans-fat. Olive oil, avocado oil, butter, and ghee (clarified butter) (see recipes in Chapter Twelve) may also be used, but canola oil and any form of margarine should be completely avoided.

In addition, you should consume either high-quality cod liver oil (for correct dosage, see Chapter Nine) and/or ground flaxseeds daily to assure adequate levels of these vital nutrients. In Chapter Nine, I'll reveal the best sources and correct doses of these supplements, as dictated by your body weight and other factors.

Oils to Avoid

Omega-6 and omega-3 are considered essential fats, but nearly all of us have an excess of omega-6 fat due to our consumption of grains and grain-raised animals. Anthropological nutritionists tell us that Paleolithic man had a ratio of omega 6:3 of approximately 1:1. And that may be still optimal. The Japanese, currently the longest-lived people, have a ratio of 3:1, which some experts consider the best ratio. However, ours is 15:1. To balance *your* ratio, eat more omega-3 fats, and fewer omega-6 fats. When you follow my dietary recommendations, you'll be doing just that, so you don't have to go out looking for omega-3 fats. Rest assured that eating the right fats won't increase your insulin levels. However, if you eat excessive omega-6 fats from processed vegetable oils, you'll alter your omega fats ratio, and contribute to weight gain.

First, eliminate most commercial vegetable oils, high in omega-6 oils, such as corn oil, safflower oil, sunflower oil, and sesame oil. Canola oil is an even less healthy choice.

Trans-Fats

Avoid all partially hydrogenated vegetable oils, which are a form of dangerous trans-fatty acids. Contained in products like margarine, Crisco, commercial mayonnaise and salad dressing, Cool Whip, commercial corn and hydrogenated oils like Wesson and others, these are poison to your system and must be strictly avoided. Products like doughnuts, crackers, cookies, pastries, deep-fat fried foods (including those from all major "fast-food" chains), potato and corn chips, imitation cheese, frosting, and candies often contain them. With nearly 100% trans-fatty acids, commercially prepared French fries are one of the most toxic foods you can eat.

Butter vs. Margarine

On all phases of this diet, you will consume butter and ghee (clarified butter used in cooking) (see recipes in Chapter Twelve). A rich source of vitamin A, which helps maintain your vision and balance your hormonal system, butter contains many other valuable vitamins (E, K, and D), as well as butyric acid, an anticarcinogen, used to build energy. Steer clear of all vegetable oil margarines, as even those made without trans-fats have been heated to extremely high temperatures, which can cause health problems.

In descending order of quality, here are my recommendations on butter:

Optimally, purchase raw butter, produced from grass-fed cows.

Second choice, organic butter, obtainable from your health food store.

Third, any store-bought butter.

Margarine is not allowed on this diet.

Avoid Sugar

The most acceptable sweetener is raw honey, which is solid at room temperature, as it has never been heated above 105 degrees. Raw honey still has all of its live enzymes, which help your body digest it.

Refined sugar weakens your immune system and promotes yeast overgrowth. All non-diet sodas contain eight teaspoons of sugar in each can. Most packaged cereals list sugar as their major ingredient. Avoid them!

When in doubt about the sugar content of a food, look at the list of ingredients to check the number of grams of carbohydrates. Unless these carbohydrates come from aboveground vegetables (such as zucchini or tomatoes), they function like sugars to alter your insulin levels.

Sweeteners

During Start-Up and Stabilize, also avoid most natural sweeteners (including corn syrup, fructose, honey, sucrose, maltodextrin, dextrose, molasses, rice milk, almond milk, white grape juice, sweetened fruit juice, brown rice syrup, maple syrup, date sugar, cane sugar, corn sugar, beet sugar, sucanat, and lactose).

If you are overweight, you have likely trained your hormone system to respond to sweets. As soon as anything sweet hits your mouth, even a low-calorie natural sweetener like stevia, your body will instantly release insulin—even though it's unnecessary. This reaction is similar to the famed response of Pavlov's dogs, who learned to salivate at the ringing of a bell, which they associated with receiving food. On the

No-Grain Diet, your taste buds will be reeducated by omitting sweets for several weeks. Take this opportunity to explore the use of spices and fresh organic food. You'll be surprised to find that foods taste better than ever.

If you are following the Booster or Core Food Plans, once you get to Sustain, you may use minimal portions of the following, healthier natural sweeteners: honey, rice syrup, beet sugar, maple syrup, and molasses. While you may use raw honey and maple syrup (in limited amounts) to prepare desserts (see recipes in Chapter Twelve), that doesn't mean you should make it a practice to pour either of them in your tea or all over your pancakes, because if you do, you'll stimulate an insulin surge. The *No-Grain Diet* has reeducated your physiology and taste buds, so please take care not to revert to old harmful habits. For those on the Advanced Food Plan, once you get to Sustain, fruits are the only acceptable dessert.

No Artificial Sweeteners

Equal and most other artificial sweeteners need to be eliminated. There are more adverse reactions to NutraSweet reported to the FDA than all other foods and additives combined. In certain individuals, it can have devastating consequences. I do not recommend the herb stevia as a sweetener either, since it can stimulate addictive sugar cravings.

Salt

Since the body needs a basic amount of sodium to function properly, most people are actually *harmed* by very low-salt diets. Common table salt contains chemical additives and is processed at over 1200 degrees, which changes its chemical structure, and, therefore, it should not be used often. Unprocessed sea salts work better with your body. Used liberally on greens, like kale, salt can decrease their bitterness. If you need to avoid salt due to high blood pressure or kidney problems, lemon crystals and lemon pepper are good replacements, giving your food a mouthwatering zing.

No-Grain Diet Foods to Eliminate

All grain products

All desserts, including cakes, cookies, candies, ice cream, muffins, and puddings

All sweeteners and sugars, including aspartame (NutraSweet or Equal) and sucralose (Splenda)

Sodas, coffee, tea, colas, diet drinks, fruit juices

Trans-fatty acids (in baked goods and all fried foods and margarine)

MSG and all artificial preservatives and chemicals

Sweetened condiments, like ketchup, pickles, and barbecue sauce

---

What Can I Drink?

In the Booster Food Plan, you can have coffee and tea. However, because it can cause complications, caffeine should be avoided by all pregnant women. On the Core Food Plan, you will eliminate it since it raises your cholesterol, worsens your insulin levels, contributes to rheumatoid arthritis and stroke, damages your blood vessels, increases the risk of heart disease, and also contributes to miscarriage. While in transition into the diet, you can continue to drink it, cutting back gradually. On the Core Food Plan you must be actively stopping, and once your are on the Advanced Food Plan it's time to quit. Coffee should never be consumed if you are pregnant or have high blood pressure, insomnia, or anxiety.

On all Food Plans, avoid sodas, sports drinks, and fruit juices, which contain refined carbohydrates and mold. The best drink is water and, in the next chapter I will explain more about its benefits as well as the pros and cons of different kinds of water and water filtration systems.

Alcohol

Eliminate all forms of alcohol—beer, wine, and hard liquor—until Sustain, when red wine is acceptable once you have reached your goal weight. People with liver disease or a history of alcohol abuse should not drink at all.

Condiments

Avoid ketchup, barbecue sauce, sweet pickles, fast-food "sauces," and sandwich spreads, as they contain added sugar. Mayonnaise and mustard are fine. Use grape-seed-oil mayonnaise from the health food store, or make your own using the recipe in Chapter Twelve. You can also make your own *No-Grain Ketchup* without added sweeteners, and you'll find a recipe in Chapter Twelve.

In Chapter Nine, I will introduce you to exercise, lifestyle changes, and supplements that amplify the impact of the *No-Grain Diet*. Remember to consult Chapter Eight for Menu Plans and Chapter Twelve for a selection of the delicious recipes you can enjoy on this diet.

CHAPTER 8

MENU PLANS

When starting the *No-Grain Diet,* some of my patients check out the allowed food lists and only see all the foods they'll be eliminating. But once I show them the sample menu plans, they all get excited by the variety and quantity of delicious and healthy food choices that are allowed on this diet. These menus help fulfill my promise that you'll never be hungry. All it takes is some planning. I advise you to sit down with pen and paper and make a weekly menu plan and shopping list. That way, you will be certain to have on hand all the foods you need.

To help you, in this chapter I've provided a full week's menu plans for each of the three Food Plans: Booster, Core, and Advanced. These plans can be used for both Start-Up and Stabilize phases of the diet. During Start-Up, you'll also need additional snacks since you'll be eating every two hours. The Creative Snack Ideas later in this chapter will provide a wide range of options for supplementing your menu plan for the first three days you're in Start-Up.

Now that you've decided which of the three Food Plans—Booster, Core, or Advanced—you'll follow, consult the Menu Plan and use it as a base for food choices and menus that are appropriate. In creating these menu plans, I've emphasized the healthiest food choices, so there are many dishes that can be used on all of the Food Plans. However, on the Booster Food Plan, I've also included a few meals that contain foods I don't consider premium, such as seafood, tofu, and dairy products, just to give you a sense of when and how often to include them. If you are on either the Core or Advanced Food Plan, you will avoid those foods.

I urge you to stay within the approved *No-Grain Diet* food guidelines while emphasizing foods you like. In Chapter Twelve I am providing a sampling of recipes, but please add other ones you know. Search cookbooks, the Internet, and *www.nograindiet.com* for additional recipes and food ideas. The recipe section contains mostly ones you might have difficulty locating elsewhere, such as my *No-Grain Pasta* recipes. As a result, to prepare more common recipes you will find on the menu plan, such as hamburgers or roasted turkey, you will need to consult other sources. In addition, you may wish to adjust your menu plans to the season. While I provide a cross-section of cool and warm recipes, you may wish to emphasize raw juices, soups, dips, and salads in warmer weather, and eat heartier cooked foods and soups when the temperature drops.

Following the Plan

Remember that anyone on the Booster Food Plan can eat all foods and meals recommended on the two higher plans, while anyone on the Core Food Plan can eat foods on the Core and Advanced Food Plans. Since the Advanced Food Plan contains the most restricted food choices, if you're on it you will need to be more careful in selecting meal options from the other two plans, as well as from other cookbooks. Study the ingredients and you'll see that many recipes will also be appropriate for you. Just check to make sure that you are using only foods on your allowed lists. This advice applies to all Food Plans. If you find that any recipe (recommended here or from other sources) contains an ingredient not allowed on your diet, decide whether you can either omit that ingredient or find a substitute. If not, find another recipe.

For example, let's say you're on the Advanced Food Plan and you find a recipe for a tofu dish. Tofu is not on your plan. You could decide to substitute chicken or tempeh. Or say you find a delicious cookbook recipe for beef stew, but it contains root vegetables like carrots and potatoes, not allowed during Start-Up and Stabilize phases of the Diet. You might choose to simply remove them from the recipe, or you could substitute another vegetable, like Brussels sprouts.

Be creative and feel free to adapt ideas you find here and elsewhere to meet your dietary requirements. In the menu plans (later in this chapter) you will find many creative ideas you can use as a starting point.

Fine-Tuning Your Meals

Remember, the menu plans provide you with basic guidelines, which you can fine-tune to create varied meals, optimal for you. As you get a sense of your personal fuel mix (see "How to Find Your Personal Fuel Mix" in Chapter Five), you can adjust the serving sizes accordingly, choosing larger or smaller portions of proteins and vegetables depending on your own needs. If you're cooking for your family, different family members with different nutritional needs can all enjoy optimal nutrition on the same menu plan if you adjust individual serving sizes of protein and vegetables to assure that all are well nourished.

Taste and experiment. Pay attention to how you feel after meals. Does a heavy protein meal leave you feeling energized? Or groggy? Adjust your fuel mix accordingly. Are you getting enough to eat at snacks? Or does the amount of meals and snacks feel overwhelming? Always feel free to eat a little more, or a little less, to find what's right for you.

On the diet, you will be eating healthy quantities of vegetables, some of them raw, to avoid ketosis. If you are unaccustomed to preparing vegetables, you will find some useful recipes in Chapter Twelve. Following my recipes, you'll learn how to juice, stir-fry, and create high-energy, high-protein raw soups and drinks. In addition, consult cookbooks and my website for recipes for salads, steamed vegetables, and other basics for incorporating more vegetables into your diet.

Another important ingredient in optimal nutrition is eating the *right kinds* of proteins—and that too is highly individual. In Chapter Five, when you took the Quick Metabolic Profile Quiz, you may have noticed that your protein preferences helped determine how you should follow the diet. Some people find red meats, like beef or lamb, and organ meats, like liver, too heavy to digest. They prefer the taste and feel better eating lighter proteins, like poultry and fish. Others don't feel satisfied without the heavier meats. And some of us are somewhere in between.

Based on the principles derived from the nutritional system I use (called Metabolic Typing), I always encourage people to go with what feels right in their protein choices. Your tastes and preferences reflect your body's wisdom. They are signals your body sends to tell you what your metabolism requires to produce energy optimally.

For example, if at Thanksgiving you always prefer a specific type of turkey meat, either dark or white, your body is giving you a useful clue. These meats differ in the types of amino acids and fat content they provide. Your body may "know" what you require. So if a dish calls for the chicken breast and you prefer the leg, adjust accordingly. If you tend to prefer lamb to chicken, feel free to make the delicious curry recipe you will find in Chapter Twelve with lamb. Conversely, if you have a profound aversion to dark meat—if even thinking of steak makes you nauseous because it sits in your stomach, avoid using beef in the recipes as this protein is too difficult for you to break down. You will need to substitute lighter-weight proteins like white meat, fish, eggs, or allowable dairy proteins.

Any of the recipes provided or menu options suggested can be prepared with a different choice of protein source. In developing your menu plans, always tune in to your natural tastes and follow them. Within each recipe there is considerable "room to move"—you are not bound to stick to its exact ingredients, proportions, or flavorings, and should feel free to modify it. That's why you will find that many recipes I offer contain variations. That way, once you master the recipe, it will be simpler to prepare it different ways or to change it by adding ingredients you like.

Stocking Up

In addition, I encourage you to try new meats, such as bison and ostrich, to provide variety to your taste buds and increase nutritional value. In order to have adequate supplies of the foods you will need for the varied meals and frequent snacks on the Diet, prepare additional food quantities, freeze them, and thaw them when needed. It's helpful to have on hand sliced turkey, beef, and chicken, and small servings of ground beef, turkey, and bison that you can use to make soups, chilies, roll-ups, and other snack foods. Soup stocks can be frozen and then used in different recipes. The sausage recipe can be prepared in advance and frozen. Raw vegetables can be cleaned, sliced, and stored so that they are ready for use. Other food preparation tips can cut meal preparation time. Keep an olive oil and lemon juice salad dressing on hand. Beans and lentils can be soaked overnight, drained, and cooked during the day in a slow cooker.

It's ideal to cook meals you can enjoy over several days, or to spend some time before your workday preparing the foods you'll cook for dinner, to shorten preparation time when you return home from work. Sometimes waiting for a meal to cook can trigger nibbling. Keep chopped raw vegetables on hand for meal prep munchies. Learn the art of staying well nourished.

Enjoying the *No-Grain Diet*

What to Eat for Breakfast

Eggs, stuffed peppers, turkey bacon, and tomato on romaine leaves, and other savory dishes for which I'll provide recipes, make excellent breakfasts. Freshly made vegetable juice and certain brands of protein drinks are an energizing way to start the day. One cornerstone of my food plan is eating high quantities of vegetables, and these are most easily incorporated through salads, juices, and certain protein drinks. In the recipe chapter, I'll provide guidelines about what to juice and what not to juice, as well as things you can add to your breakfast vegetable juice (or use instead of juicing if your time is limited) to increase your vitality.

**Five Breakfast Ideas
(Booster, Core, Advanced)**

1. Poached eggs over salmon hollandaise on a bed of steamed spinach

2. *Dr. Mercola's Basic Green Drink** with *Turkey and Cheese Roll-Ups**

3. *No-Grain Pancakes** with *Cinnamon Butter** and *Mediterranean Sausage Patty**

4. *Italian Sausage Patty** with *Tomato-Thyme Quiche,** topped with sprouts.

5. *No-Grain Bread** with tahini spread served with walnut-flax whey protein shake.

---

*Recipes can be found in Chapter Twelve.

I consider vegetable juice one of the best ways to incorporate large quantities of raw foods, which contain chlorophyll and phytonutrients, into your diet. I am convinced that this is one of the most powerful tools one can use to obtain high-level vitality. I see many seriously ill patients and I am always amazed at the potency of vegetable juice in restoring their health and energy levels. For many of us, compromised digestive function limits the ability to absorb nutrients from vegetables. Juicing (or the use of certain high-quality protein drinks) helps to deliver nutrients "predigested" for you.

If you are not yet ready to advance into juicing, use a protein shake (see Protein Powder recommendations earlier in this chapter and in the Appendix) along with some fish oil (see Chapter Nine for dosage). You may also enjoy a side dish of fresh or cooked vegetables. For convenience I recommend a high-quality protein drink. For further information at *www.nograindiet.com*.

What to Eat for Snacks

Follow these tips to get the best value from your snacks:

- Vary your snacks so that you get both nourishment and real enjoyment from them.

- Always have extra snacks on hand, so that you're never tempted to reach for a candy bar or other wrong foods.
- Keep a mini-blender and recommended protein powder at work to make protein drinks for times when unexpected hunger pangs hit.
- Keep hard-boiled eggs, sliced vegetables, cherry tomatoes, or other favorite snack foods on hand in your home and work fridge for a ready snack.
- Use protein leftovers to make roll-ups, a delicious way to combine meat and vegetables. (See recipes in Chapter Twelve.)
- Raw energy soups (flavored in different ways) can be made in a blender or Cuisinart. Easy to prepare, they deliver raw vegetables in a tasty and easy to digest form. (See recipes in Chapter Twelve.)
- Raw coconut slices are also an excellent snack choice.

How to Open a Coconut

Organic coconuts taste better because they are not irradiated. To prepare, pierce two of the three eyes with an ice pick and drain the coconut juice. Or you can use a small Phillips screwdriver and a hammer. Crack open the shell with the hammer, aiming for a ridge at the eye end. Break the meat from the shell, and scrape or peel the dark inner skin away from the flesh with a strong knife, being careful to point it away from your other hand.

Once you have removed the chunks of coconut, please note the color and texture. The coconut meat should be bright white, firm, and tasty. If it is soft, moldy, or odd tasting, please throw it away, as it may be too old. The backing behind the white coconut should be a smooth, unbroken homogenous dark brown. If patches of white come through, the coconut is too old to eat. Also, that brown backing can be eaten. It does not have to be peeled off.

Coconut can be eaten in chunks, grated, toasted, or blended with water to prepare coconut milk, an excellent ingredient for smoothies, soups, and gravies.

I'll guarantee you'll find it's easy to adapt to more frequent meals. Feel free to select from my Creative Snacks Ideas below, or use your own favorites. Prepare your snacks to bring with you to work, so you always have them on hand. Check out nearby restaurants, salad bars, diners, or snack bars for grain-free soups and salads to add to snack foods you bring from home.

---

40 Creative Snack Ideas

- *Dr. Mercola's Basic Green Drink with protein powder**
- Goat cheese with vegetable plate
- Fresh coconut chunks
- *Chicken Roll-Ups** with chopped salad
- Raw basil tomato soup with choice of meat/poultry
- *Mushroom-Chicken Quiche** with small salad
- Chilled raw cucumber soup with choice of meat/poultry
- Goat yogurt with cinnamon-walnut crumble
- Protein shake with crudités and walnut butter
- Avocado dip, veggies, and choice of meat/poultry
- Shrimp cocktail with cocktail sauce of *No-Grain Ketchup** and horseradish
- Vegetable pâté, veggies, and choice of meat/poultry
- *Cream of Vegetable Soup** with choice of meat/poultry
- Sardines with *Multicolored Slaw**
- *Raw Ginger Energy Soup** with choice of meat or tempeh
- French onion soup (without the bread) with choice of meat/poultry
- *Beef Roll-Ups** with horseradish dressing
- Miso soup with scallions and choice of meat/poultry
- Grape leaves stuffed with choice of meat/poultry
- *Creamy Fish Cakes** with *Lemon-Dill Mayonnaise**
- Celery stuffed with *Hummus,** or walnut or pumpkin seed butter
- Stuffed pepper with choice of meat/poultry, salad, or chili
- Fruit protein smoothie
- *Oven Kohlrabi Crisps** with choice of meat/poultry
- *Tandoori Kabobs** with choice of meat/poultry
- Raw apple with cheese or nut butter
- Cod bites with seafood sauce
- Vegetable soup au gratin with "mini-meatballs"
- Boston lettuce salad with choice of meat/poultry

- *Italian Sausage Quiche**
- Endive and raw tahini with flax-berry smoothie (Sustain only)
- Broccoli frittata
- *Jerk Sausage Patty** "sandwich" between two thick slices of tomato*
- Sliced turkey and cheese with grilled peppers and salsa
- Hard-boiled eggs with mayo and radishes
- Zucchini stuffed with meat hash
- "Mini-burgers" with fixings and *No-Grain Ketchup**
- *Creamy Cheese and Vegetable Soup** with meat slices.
- Turkey Bacon "LT"
- Broiled sesame tofu

*Recipes can be found in Chapter Twelve.

What to Eat for Lunch

If you can, make your own lunch and avoid restaurants. A salad with some meat is a good all-purpose meal.

5 Lunch Ideas

1. Buffalo burger with *No-Grain Ketchup**, tomato slices, and red onion; watercress and greens salad with Roquefort dressing

2. *Asian Turkey Salad** on bed of dandelion greens with ginger-scallion dressing; steamed garlic green beans

3. *Southwestern Beef Chili** with grated cheddar served over steamed broccoli spears with melted butter; green salad with walnut-parsley dressing

4. Open-faced grass-fed beef with *Gravy** served over *No-Grain Bread**; Boston lettuce with bean sprouts salad seasoned with Russian dressing

5. *Pinto bean/Chicken Roll-Ups,** served with salsa, guacamole, organic sour cream, and shredded goat cheddar

*Recipes can be found in Chapter Twelve.

Do-It-Yourself Salad

Pour salad dressing made with extra-virgin olive oil into a wide-mouthed quart Mason or Ball jar.

Add a serving of chicken, turkey, beef, or eggs.
Add hot peppers, like giardiniera, sliced onion, chopped garlic, or olives.
Add sliced peppers, mushrooms, or tomatoes.
Add mixed greens, sliced vegetables, and chopped herbs.

The meat acts as a barrier between the dressing and the vegetables, keeping them nice and fresh. When you empty the jar, the dressing will be on top of the salad just as it should be.

Restaurant Eating the *No-Grain Diet* Way

If you eat regularly in restaurants, the following simple guidelines help:

- Try Chinese, Indian, Thai, and other ethnic cuisines, where you can order meat and vegetable dishes, but make sure to pass on the rice and noodles.
- At Italian restaurants, sidestep the pasta in favor of chicken, meat, or seafood dishes with vegetable sides.
- Seek out homemade soups at local delis, diners, and soup bars, where you can request a serving with more broth, and bypass noodles, rice, and potatoes added to soups. (It's okay to take them out with your spoon if you have to!)
- Always move the bread and rolls away from your side of the table, or ask the waiter to remove them altogether.
- Order a salad, served with lemon slices and olive oil on the side, to bypass goopy dressings made with undesirable oils.
- Ask for salad or vegetable side dishes in place of fries, pasta, or potatoes.
- Order an appetizer, if necessary, in addition to the entrée, to ensure you are well nourished and not tempted by dessert (and coffee, to be eliminated later on in the Diet).

- Keep packets of herbal tea with you to have in place of after-meal coffees and caffeinated teas.

Best Soup Choices

Chili
Chunky tomato
Creamy Vegetable Soup*
French onion soup with cheese (minus the bread)
Mushroom soup (no barley)
Thai chicken coconut
Miso soup
Egg-drop soup
Energy Soup*
Lemongrass soup
Minestrone (minus the pasta)
Mulligatawny
Split pea
Lentil
Fish or clam chowder (minus potatoes)
Chicken with matzo ball (minus the matzo ball)

And remember, no crackers. If you still feel hungry, eat turkey slices, a burger, a side of cooked vegetables, or a salad.

---

*Recipes can be found in Chapter Twelve.

Ten Recipes

To maintain a successful diet over the long term, it's important to find ten recipes that really work for you. I learned this bit of wisdom early in my medical training, from Dr. William P. Castelli, M.D., director of the Framingham Heart Study, who noted, after evaluating five thousand people for nearly three decades, that "Most people only rotate through ten different recipes throughout their lives. [After trying] different meals, they seem to settle on ten meals they routinely consume."

In my practice, I have confirmed his observation. However, some people routinely use *fewer* recipes, which makes it tougher to implement the Diet. If that's true for you, I encourage you to explore and experiment until you find ten recipes you really like, even if you end up trying forty or fifty recipes to find them. Start by trying the menu plans and recipes I offer here, and you will find a great support for your weight loss and ongoing health.

Using the Menu Plans

Use the Sample Start-Up Menu Plan as a model to plan the meals and snacks you will eat during Start-Up. Consult the Sample Start-Up Shopping List to get an idea of the groceries you would need to buy if you were to follow the sample, and make a shopping list of items you will need to have on hand for the meals *you* plan to eat during Start-Up. If you know you'll be obtaining certain food items at a restaurant near work, for example, note that on your shopping list, so that all necessary foods are accounted for.

Sample Start-Up Menu Plan			
	Day 1	Day 2	Day 3
7 A.M. BREAKFAST	Poached eggs hollandaise over spinach topped with turkey bacon	*Leek-Bacon-Garlic Quiche* with fried green tomatoes and *Mediterranean Sausage Patty*	Turkey hash with poached eggs and *No-Grain Ketchup*
9 A.M. SNACK	*Hummus* with cucumber	Chunky coconut protein drink	*No-Grain Walnut Muffin* with walnut butter
11 A.M. SNACK	Lentil soup with Swiss cheese topping	Turkey chunks with crudités and cilantro dipping sauce	*Mint Watercress Energy Soup* with protein powder
1 P.M. LUNCH	Veal Piccata with garlic green beans and Caesar salad	Creamy cod with baked garlic mushrooms, green salad with shallot vinaigrette	Grass-fed beef cheeseburger and *Mexican Coleslaw* with baked turnip slices

	Day 1	Day 2	Day 3
3 P.M. SNACK	Salmon salad stuffed in a tomato	Veal hash in a green pepper	Yogurt with coconut walnut crunch
5 P.M. SNACK	*Cream of Vegetable Soup** with *Jerk Sausage Patty**	*Creamy Fish Cakes** with crisp veggies	Beef slices with chunky salsa
7 P.M. DINNER	Roast turkey with cranberry salsa, served with spinach salad with lemon mint dressing and baked cauliflower	*Pepper steak** with *Stir-Fried Vegetables**	Crisp organic duck served with buttery Brussels sprouts and a mixed green salad
9 P.M. SNACK	*Turkey/Spinach Roll-Ups** with cranberry salsa	*Creamy Asparagus soup**	Turkey vegetable soup with *Kohlrabi Crisps**

* Recipes can be found in Chapter Twelve.

Sample Start-Up Shopping List

Meat, Fish, Poultry (organic and grass-
    fed preferred)
Beef, ground
Bison, ground
Chicken
Cod
Duck
Flank steak
Ostrich, ground
Salmon
Turkey, whole
Turkey bacon

Dairy Products (organic preferred)
Butter
Cheese: Swiss, cheddar
Cream, heavy
Eggs
Parmesan cheese
Yogurt: whole milk, plain

Spices, Herbs, Condiments
Apple cider vinegar
Celtic salt
Chives
Cinnamon, ground
Coconut, unsweetened, grated
Dill
Garlic powder
Ginger, ground or fresh root
Mint
Mustard powder
Parsley
Thyme

Protein Powders
Choice of:
Whey protein
Rice protein

(continued)

Miscellaneous
Anchovies
Chicken broth
Natural mustard
Salsa
Sardines
Wheat-free tamari soy sauce

Vegetables (organic preferred)
Asparagus
Brussels sprouts
Cabbage
Cauliflower
Celery
Cilantro
Cucumbers
Garlic
Green beans
Green pepper
Kale
Kohlrabi
Lettuce: Boston, green leaf, mesclun,
    romaine
Mesclun mixed greens
Mint, fresh
Onions

Radicchio
Scallions
Shallots
Shiitaki and white mushrooms
Spinach
Sprouts
Tomatoes
Turnips
Watercress
Zucchini

Fruit
Avocados
Cranberries
Lemon
Orange

Nuts, Seeds, Oils
Coconut oil, organic
Flaxseeds, raw, organic
Olive oil, organic, cold-pressed
Walnuts, raw, organic

Legumes (dried beans)
Chickpeas
Lentils

In planning your meals, you may also consult the Stabilize Menu Plans, later in this chapter, and the Creative Snack Ideas, earlier in this chapter. The one-week Stabilize Menu Plans can serve as a guide for both Start-Up and Stabilize. The only difference between the first two phases is that during Start-Up, you eat every two hours. In 40 Creative Snack Ideas (page 129), you'll find additional snacks you can adopt and add to your menu plan while you are in Start-Up.

Booster Food Plan: Start-Up and Stabilize Menu Plan

	MONDAY	TUESDAY	WEDNESDAY	THURSDAY	FRIDAY	SATURDAY	SUNDAY
BREAKFAST	Scrambled tofu with corned beef hash and No-Grain Ketchup*	Deviled eggs over Boston lettuce salad with bacon and avocado slices	Spinach-feta omelette with grilled tomatoes topped with melted cheese	Grapefruit slices Italian Sausage Quiche*	Turkey bacon LT with Multicolored Cole Slaw*	No-Grain Pancakes* and Cinnamon Butter* Mediterranean Sausage Patty*	Salmon/goat cheese omelette Sprout/watercress salad
A.M. SNACK	Creamy Mushroom Soup* and turkey slices	Green Drink with protein powder* and Swiss cheese slices	Thai chicken soup with fresh coconut chunks	Yogurt with cinnamon apple sauce	Cream of Asparagus Soup* and spicy chicken leg/breast	Scoop of cottage cheese and red pepper slices	Creamy Cheddar Broccoli Soup* with Italian Sausage Patty*
LUNCH	Orange beef and Stir-Fried Vegetables*	Balsamic chicken breast over Caesar salad	Grass-fed burger, turnip fries and No-Grain Ketchup* Mexican Coleslaw*	Cobb salad Grilled garlic zucchini, parsley vinaigrette	Ham/cheddar soufflé with creamed spinach	Southwestern Buffalo Chili,* mesclun salad, miso dressing Baked kohlrabi	Open-faced beef with Gravy* over No-Grain Bread* with Boston lettuce with bean sprouts salad
P.M. SNACK	Hummus* and cauliflower bites Rice protein drink	Lentil soup and grilled chicken leg/breast	No-Grain Muffin* with goat cheese and celery sticks	Miso soup with tofu and seaweed salad	Chef salad with Russian dressing Grilled vegetables	Red pepper stuffed with chicken salad	Tomato vegetable soup and crispy turkey wing/breast
DINNER	Greek lamb moussaka Greek salad Steamed Swiss chard	German sauerbraten Turnip fries Red cabbage with caraway	Creamy baked cod with steamed broccoli and green salad, mustard vinaigrette	Italian Zucchini "Lasagna"* with Meat Sauce* and mixed salad	Bombay Chicken Curry* with red lentil dal and cucumber raita.	Pepper Steak* and broccoli with garlic sauce Asian Slaw*	Roast turkey, Brussels sprouts, baked turnips, cranberry salsa
SNACK	Apple slices and walnut butter, miso, and raw cheddar	Red cabbage and beef strips	Creamy Fish Cake* with Dill-Lemon Mayonnaise*	Italian Sausage Patty* with mixed salad	Cranberry protein drink	Shrimp with No-Grain Ketchup* and horseradish cocktail sauce	Turkey Roll-Up* with sprouts and tomato

Core Food Plan: Start-Up and Stabilize Menu Plan

	MONDAY	TUESDAY	WEDNESDAY	THURSDAY	FRIDAY	SATURDAY	SUNDAY
BREAKFAST	Poached eggs and salmon hollandaise over spinach	Mushroom omelette Creamed broccoli Jerk Sausage Patty*	Leek-Bacon-Garlic Quiche*	Melted cheddar with sun-dried tomatoes on No-Grain Toast* with protein drink	Baked eggs with beef hash, grilled onions and No-Grain Ketchup*	Mexican scrambled eggs with refried beans, salsa, and sour cream	Dr. Mercola's Green Drink* Ratatouille with refried beans, and Italian Beef Sausage Patty*
A.M. SNACK	Miso soup and crisp tempeh/chicken	Onion soup with Swiss cheese topping, beef mini-burgers	Mediterranean Sausage Patty* with Multicolored Coleslaw*	Leek-Bacon-Garlic Quiche*	Turkey Roll-Ups* with Avocado Mayonnaise* and endive	Midsummer Gazpacho Energy Soup* and celery with bean dip	Raw Garlic Energy Soup* with walnuts and coconut chunks
LUNCH	Beef Tandoori Kabobs* Spinach salad with shredded radish and Dijon vinaigrette	Asian Chicken Salad* on bed of greens Steamed garlic green beans	Halibut Fish Cake* with Lemon-Dill Mayonnaise* and mixed green salad	Confetti Pasta with Walnut Pesto* and meatballs with green salad	Buffalo burger Grilled portobello mushroom with goat cheese Watercress/greens salad	Southwestern Tempeh Chili* and Mexican Cole Slaw*	Poached salmon over endive, spinach, radicchio salad/mustard vinaigrette
P.M. SNACK	Hummus* with chopped tomato-cake salad	Raw Avocado-Cucumber Soup with Turkey Roll-Ups*	Egg-drop soup Steak strips with ginger sauce	Duck Roll-Ups* with Roasted Garlic Miso Sauce*	Avocado half with cottage cheese	Baked garlic mushrooms stuffed with turkey hash	Mushroom-Chicken Quiche* with grilled endive
DINNER	Chicken parmigiana, broccolini and tri-color salad	Baked halibut, broccoli au gratin, salad and peppercorn dressing	Veal Stew* with baked turnips, kale salad	Dijon lamb chops with Braised Brussels sprouts	Thai Chicken Curry* Spinach with chick-peas and sprout salad	Grass-fed meat loaf, Cauliflower Mashers with Gravy,* green salad with lemon-dill dressing	Pepper Steak* Mixed steamed greens with Arugala Pesto* and green salad
SNACK	Coconut rice protein shake	Beef shiitake mushroom soup	Tamari walnuts and whey protein shake	Coconut Yogurt Smoothie	Asparagus Leek Soup* with Thai chicken chunks	Beef Roll-Ups* with Sundried Tomato Pesto*	Hummus* with fennel

Advanced Food Plan: Start-Up and Stabilize Menu Plan

	MONDAY	TUESDAY	WEDNESDAY	THURSDAY	FRIDAY	SATURDAY	SUNDAY
BREAKFAST	Dr. Mercola's Basic Green Drink* or poached eggs with Thai Sausage Patty*	Dr. Mercola's Basic Green Drink* or Chicken Roll-Ups*	Dr. Mercola's Basic Green Drink* or portobello mushroom stuffed with buffalo pâté	Dr. Mercola's Basic Green Drink* or scrambled tempeh and Jerk Sausage Patty*	Dr. Mercola's Basic Green Drink* or No-Grain Pancakes* with turkey bacon	Dr. Mercola's Basic Green Drink* or salmon with Lemon-Dill Mayonnaise*	Dr. Mercola's Basic Green Drink* with rice protein or curried egg salad over No-Grain Toast*
A.M. SNACK	Dr. Mercola's Basic Green Drink* or celery, fennel, cucumber juice and coconut, and rice protein drink	Dr. Mercola's Basic Green Drink* or red leaf, spinach, celery juice with cranberries, and rice protein shake	Dr. Mercola's Basic Green Drink* or celery, cucumber, spinach, escarole, fennel, and whey protein drink	Ginger Energy Soup* with chunks of coconut	Dr. Mercola's Basic Green Drink* or romaine, endive, celery, parsley, ginger, and whey protein drink	Dr. Mercola's Basic Green Drink* or green leaf, celery, lemon, and rice protein drink	Dr. Mercola's Basic Green Drink* or Gazpacho Energy Soup*
LUNCH	Lamb Stew* with green beans and tomato salad	Asian Beef Salad* over baby greens Steamed asparagus	Pinto bean and chicken "burrito" with leaf lettuce "taco" and trimmings	Curried chicken salad over cuke/watercress salad with mint dressing	Salmon Cakes* with Avocado Mayonnaise* Steamed asparagus, vegetable salad and raspberry vinaigrette	Southwestern Beef Chili* with broccoli spears Green salad with walnut dressing	Buffalo mushroom Bourguignon, Mesclun salad vinaigrette
P.M. SNACK	Organic chopped liver with hearts of lettuce and red onion slices	Creamy Broccoli Soup* with Jerk Sausage Patty*	Sardines with Multicolored Slaw*	Beef Roll-Ups* with Wasabi Dip*	Salmon and mustard sauce rolled in romaine leaves	Chilled raw cucumber bisque with grass-fed steak bits	Pepper stuffed with beef chili Cucumber rounds
DINNER	Garlic grass-fed pot roast, with zucchini, onions Tomato salad	Thai Chicken Curry* with scallion/ginger bok choy and sprouts salad	Filet mignon with Stir-Fried Vegetables* roasted turnips	Broiled wild salmon, marinated cauliflower, and broccoli salad	Lemon-roasted Cornish hens Endive salad with vinaigrette walnut asparagus	Zucchini "Lasagna"* with Tomato Meat Sauce* and Caesar salad	Roast leg of lamb, green beans and mixed vegetable salad with mint dressing
SNACK	Pot roast slices with horseradish and tomatoes	Tamari walnuts and rice protein drink	Celery, pepper, chicken bites with Garlic Miso Dip*	Salmon salad with winter greens	Mexican Chicken Wings with guacamole and crudités	Vegetable soup with Steak Roll-Ups*	Lamb Roll-Ups* and garlic mayonnaise

Menu Plans: Sustain Phase

The following five-day menu plans will guide you in staying on the Diet during the Sustain phase. Again, there is a menu plan for each of the Food Plans: Booster, Core, and Advanced. Please make sure to first follow the guidelines in Chapter Five for a safe transition into Sustain. Once you have made that transition, and have established the correct amounts of healthy grains and starches you can safely eat, you will be ready to use the five-day menu plan. Obviously, you will be sustaining the diet for an extended period of time, so these plans are designed to give you an indication of how to incorporate healthy grains, starchy vegetables, and fruits in a safe way. You will need to locate additional recipes to continue the program. You can adjust old favorites, find new ones, and modify recipes to sustain the principles of *No-Grain* eating long-term.

Make sure to adapt these guidelines to your own needs. For example, if you have determined that you must maintain grain, starch, or fruit elimination, or severely restrict consumption, let that be your guideline in fine-tuning a menu plan customized to you. For example, for the Booster Food Plan, the Sustain menu plan contains occasional servings of fruit and healthy desserts. But if, through your transition, you have learned that you cannot eat these foods without gaining weight, or rekindling cravings, continue to eliminate them. Instead, consider increasing your level of exercise and, if you do, later monitor your consumption (as detailed in the Carb Quota Monitor on page 84) to determine whether or not you can now include occasional fruit without sacrificing your weight loss.

In Chapter Nine, I will introduce you to exercise, lifestyle changes, and supplements that amplify the impact of the *No-Grain Diet*. Remember to consult Part 4 for the delicious recipes you can enjoy on this diet.

Booster Food Plan: Sustain Menu Plan

	MONDAY	TUESDAY	WEDNESDAY	THURSDAY	FRIDAY
BREAKFAST	Italian Sausage Quiche,* raw milk cheese and tomato salad	Cheese soufflé with creamed spinach and turkey bacon	Kiwi-Strawberry Smoothie* No-Grain Walnut Muffin*	Apple-cinnamon pancakes with Chicken Sausage Patty*	Berry smoothie Tomato-Thyme Quiche*
A.M. SNACK	Pear slices and almond butter	Chicken croquette and Asian Slaw*	Sunshine Energy Soup* and deviled eggs	Tomato stuffed with turkey salad	Dr. Mercola's Basic Green Drink* or spinach cucumber, parsley, and raw cranberries juice
LUNCH	Spaghetti Squash* with Tomato Meat Sauce* and grated raw milk cheese Green salad	Creamy Halibut Fish Cakes* over raw greens with Walnut Garlic Dip* Steamed asparagus	Spinach soufflé Cauliflower au gratin Beet-endive salad	Meatball "hero" on grilled eggplant with tomato sauce and mozzarella	Salmon salad Nicoise with green beans, anchovy, and garlic dressing
P.M. SNACK	Endive and Hummus*	Melba Smoothie* with protein powder	Chicken-Asparagus Roll-Ups* with Avocado Mayonnaise*	Chopped vegetable salad with cottage cheese	Lamb Roll-Up* with Hummus* and Multicolored Slaw*
DINNER	Baked halibut Millet Pilaf* Mesclun salad and lemon poppyseed dressing	Grass-fed Beef Stew* Baked yam slices Mesclun, pear, and endive salad	Barbecued spare ribs with sautéed greens and ginger dressing Mixed sprout salad	Organic veal parmigiana and Confetti Pasta* with Walnut Pesto* Romaine salad	Asian flank steak with Stir-Fried Vegetables* and Asian Slaw*
SNACK	Mocha Meringue Cookies* with flax protein drink	Creamy Spinach Soup* with roast beef slices	Turkey slices with Basil Pesto* and crudités	Walnut Torte* with Orange Buttercream*	Carrot Zucchini Soup* with chicken breast/leg

Core Food Plan: Sustain Menu Plan

	MONDAY	TUESDAY	WEDNESDAY	THURSDAY	FRIDAY
BREAKFAST	Dr. Mercola's Basic Green Drink* or Poached egg hollandaise over spinach with Mild Sausage Patty*	Vegetable frittata Grilled zucchini and Italian Sausage Patty*	Dr. Mercola's Basic Green Drink* or Fish Nori Rolls* with Asian Ginger Sauce*	Dr. Mercola's Basic Green Drink* or No-Grain Waffle* and Mediterranean Sausage Patty*	Grapefruit Soft-boiled eggs and turkey hash
A.M. SNACK	Dr. Mercola's Basic Green Drink* or celery, fennel, cucumber and rice protein, and coconut juice	Dr. Mercola's Basic Green Drink* and grilled red pepper, feta chunks with dribbled olive oil	Autumn Harvest Energy Soup* and apples with walnut butter, miso, and raw cheddar	Dr. Mercola's Basic Green Drink* or red leaf, cabbage, celery, raw cranberries, and whey protein drink	Coconut Apricot Smoothie* with protein powder No-Grain Muffin*
LUNCH	Buffalo burgers with No-Grain Ketchup* Kohlrabi Chips* and Multicolored Coleslaw*	Poached salmon over Caesar salad Steamed asparagus hollandaise	Zucchini boats stuffed with Southwestern Turkey Chili* Parsnip and mesclun salad, lemon dressing	Cobb salad with Roquefort dressing Baked Pear* with whipped cream	Grass-fed Beef Stew* over steamed cabbage with grated carrot/sprout salad
P.M. SNACK	Spicy chicken vegetable soup, green/red pepper slices	Creamy Salmon Cake* with Lemon-Dill Mayonnaise* and celery salad	Mushroom Chicken Quiche* with grated carrot and daikon salad	Roast beef slices with horse-radish and hearts of romaine	Sardines over tossed salad with lemon-dill dressing
DINNER	Grilled lamb chops with mint-arugala salad Steamed Swiss chard	Thai Chicken Curry* with scallion/ginger bok choy	Grass-fed steak teriyaki Stir Fried Vegetables* Mixed salad with scallion dressing	Veal Marsala with broccoli rabe and mushroom brown rice risotto	Asparagus stuffed summer flounder Creamed spinach Watercress salad
SNACK	Harvest Energy Soup* with raw cheddar cheese or turkey bacon	Mexican Cole Slaw* and ginger chicken slices	Borscht topped with sour cream and hard-boiled egg	Mushroom soup with mini-burgers	No-Grain Fruit Crumble*

Advanced Food Plan: Sustain Menu Plan

	MONDAY	TUESDAY	WEDNESDAY	THURSDAY	FRIDAY
BREAKFAST	Dr. Mercola's Basic Green Drink* or celery, fennel, and cucumber juice Poached eggs over No-Grain Bread*	Dr. Mercola's Basic Green Drink* or spinach, celery, red leaf, and garlic juice Salmon Hollandaise on Millet	Dr. Mercola's Basic Green Drink* or spinach, red pepper, cheese, and turkey melt Watercress endive salad	Dr. Mercola's Basic Green Drink* or sardines and raw salsa in lettuce rolls	Dr. Mercola's Basic Green Drink* or celery, cucumber, and red leaf juice Soft-boiled eggs with Jerk Sausage Patty*
A.M. SNACK	Dr. Mercola's Basic Green Drink* or red-leaf cabbage, spinach, and ginger juice Green apple slices and walnut spread	Broccoli Energy Soup* with pumpkin seeds Buffalo Nori Roll* with Miso Sauce*	Dr. Mercola's Basic Green Drink* or cucumber, endive, bok choy, ginger, and fresh cranberries juice with rice protein powder	Dr. Mercola's Basic Green Drink* or green leaf, celery, spinach, fennel, and fresh coconut juice Grass-fed beef chili with broccoli spears	Dr. Mercola's Basic Green Drink* or cucumber, cabbage, endive, and protein drink Shiitake mushrooms stuffed with garlic tempeh
LUNCH	Coconut-crusted chicken with green salad and lemongrass flaxseed dressing Green beans	Open-faced Italian bison meatballs on No-Grain Bread* Raw zucchini salad with garlic oregano dressing	Thai Chicken Salad* over hijiki seaweed salad	Turkey Tandoori Kabobs* Spinach salad with shredded carrot and Dijon vinaigrette	Grass-fed braised short ribs of beef Saffron amaranth and mesclun salad
P.M. SNACK	Tomato basil soup, raw milk cheese stuffed mushrooms	Hummus* with crudités	Chicken salad stuffed peppers Daikon and carrot slices	Spicy cabbage beef soup	Nori Rolls* and Spicy Wasabi Sauce*
DINNER	Grass-fed buffalo meatloaf Cauliflower Mashers* Baked squash crisps	Bombay Lamb Curry* with spinach over Brown Rice* Multicolored Cole Slaw*	Walnut baked flounder on amaranth Asparagus and bean sprouts with scallion vinaigrette	Marinated grilled venison tenderloin steak Avocado, red cabbage, and red onion salad Millet Pilaf*	Roast turkey with cinnamon yams Fennel and greens salad Baked pearl onions Raw cranberry salsa
SNACK	Crunchy root and vegetable chips with garlic goat yogurt dip	Lamb kabob with coconut dipping sauce	Creamy Curry Soup* with Turkey Roll-Ups*	Flax berry whey protein shake	Autumn Harvest Energy Soup* Turkey slices

All beef recipes will work with commercial grain-fed beef, but will not be as healthy for you.
Freeze pre-cooked chicken and turkey in plastic bags for use when needed.
In the poultry recipes, choose dark or white chicken or turkey according to which is more satiating. Always cook extra protein. It will be handy for subsequent snacks and meals.
All of the italized recipes are included in Chapter Twelve.

CHAPTER 9

SUPPORTS FOR YOUR HEALTH

While the Food Plan is the foundation of my program, I want you to learn other vital factors, and integrate them into your life. I've spent decades combing the medical literature for clues to the most effective techniques, perfected their use with my patients, and created an overall program for weight loss and health, chock full of little known secrets that make a big difference in how you'll feel, look, and experience life.

Mastering lifestyle basics confers powerful health and weight-loss benefits. Things we take for granted, like drinking the right kind of water, make a difference. Obtaining restful sleep is key to your overall health. Your exposure to sun, electromagnetic fields, and light sources can strongly affect you, yet most people don't know how to extract the benefits from positive exposures and avoid the dangers of negative ones. In this chapter you'll learn how to do the right thing in all these key areas. You'll also learn the best time to quit smoking on this Diet, as well as other tips to support your health upgrade and weight loss. What's more, I've identified the most essential supplements to support your weight-loss effort.

Combining the Diet with the right exercise, supplements, and other optimal health techniques will launch you into a synergy-powered momentum toward all your goals.

Losing weight permanently and successfully requires more than changing your diet. You must change your life. Recent studies confirm three indispensable measures for reversing the insulin cycle and losing weight. I call them the Weight Loss Trio:

1. Eliminating grains, starches, and sugars
2. Exercising
3. Getting a good night's sleep

Now that you're launched the *No-Grain Diet,* let's turn our attention to the rest of the Trio. First, exercise is crucial in losing weight and in preventing diseases like heart disease and diabetes.

The Weight Loss Trio: Exercise

Exercise and Weight Loss

Major studies show that exercise prevents diseases like heart disease, cancer, and diabetes, while guaranteeing successful weight loss. Here's how: First, exercise increases your metabolic rate so that you'll burn calories even while you sleep. Second, it boosts your insulin sensitivity, decreasing insulin resistance and lowering insulin levels, making it easier to burn fat.

In exercising, remember to:

1. Listen to your body
2. Develop a consistent exercise program
3. Increase your level of exercise gradually and comfortably as your own energy increases
4. Get a personal trainer if you can, but remember to ignore his or her nutritional recommendations and use this book as your primary guide

I mention this last item because most trainers are slim, athletic folks themselves, whose advice, such as carb loading or eating sugary protein bars, is often way off base for people who need to lose weight. Respect their area of expertise, but do not make them the master of *your* nutritional destiny.

Sticking with Your Exercise Program

If you want to lose weight, you know you need to exercise. That's not new. What is new is that, thanks to EFT, it's never been easier to start and stick with an exercise program. If, in the past, you've ever had trouble staying with exercise, I encourage you to turn to the EFT chapter right now to uncover hidden feelings and beliefs and learn how to stop sabotaging yourself. With this support, you can finally start a program that will work for you.

Thirty minutes of exercise per day will deliver weight loss, while major studies indicate that sixty minutes a day (optimally continuous, or split into two sessions) is even better.

How to Begin

Start by walking and, as you become fit, increase your intensity to a level where it's mildly uncomfortable to speak while exercising. If you can comfortably chat, you aren't working hard enough to produce weight loss. If you can't speak at all, you are exercising too hard and should cut back.

Outside you can race walk. Consult *www.racewalk.com* to learn how to do that. Indoors, on a treadmill, you can raise intensity, without having to run, by increasing your incline. If you belong to a health club, use an elliptical exercise machine, which I consider the optimal aerobic exercise equipment because it provides a complete lower body workout by rotating the use of the different leg muscle groups.

Elliptical Tips

To decrease the "boredom factor," you can change the incline setting every minute or two by one notch to work different leg muscles. You can also reverse the direction of the leg movement, reducing the intensity setting one notch to make it easier. To improve your sense of balance, carefully let go of the side bars until you feel skilled and secure hands-free. Be persistent, and after a few weeks you will be quite comfortable.

Weight-bearing exercises are more effective for weight loss than non-weight-bearing exercises like swimming and bicycling, which require a much longer workout (up to four times as long!) to produce the same effect. Swimming also exposes you to large amounts of chlorine, which is absorbed through the skin. Applying olive oil immediately prior to swimming can help to decrease chlorine absorption. Swimming in a lake, river, or ocean is great.

Another useful and very inexpensive piece of equipment is a rebounder or mini-trampoline. A high-quality one that will last many years can usually be purchased for $200 to $250.

Keeping the Weight Off

Keeping the weight off is one of your biggest challenges, and this is where exercise really pays off. Research shows that exercise may normalize your body's sensitivity to the hormone leptin, which is secreted by your fat cells and helps regulate your weight.

Research Finding

In a recent animal study, researchers measured food consumption, body weight, and energy expenditure, after giving the hormone leptin to obese rats. They wanted to find out whether weight loss attained through dieting could be maintained by increased exercise. They concluded that a reduction in food intake created the initial loss of body weight; however, increased energy expenditure (folks, that means *exercise*) was key to maintaining that weight loss, and helped do so even after food consumption returned to normal.

Let me give you the bottom line here: If you fail to exercise, it's likely you'll kiss your weight loss goodbye. Exercise is critical to maintaining your weight loss during Sustain.

The Weight Loss Trio: Sleep

Subject to the pressures of modern life, many people try to gain a little extra time by reducing the hours they sleep. But that's not the way to go, because sleeping less than six and a half hours a night *increases your risk of obesity,* according to a recent study. You need at least six and a half hours, while eight hours of sleep is ideal. As you know, the three top risk factors for weight gain are *excess grain consumption, lack of exercise,* and *sleep loss.*

Turn that around and you'll see that the three most proactive steps you can take to lose weight are to eliminate grains (starches and sweets), to exercise, and yes, to sleep. That's why I want to share with you these essential steps to assuring a good night's sleep.

Sleep and Insulin

Chronic sleep deprivation increases insulin resistance exactly as aging does, a University of Chicago research team found. In their study, healthy adults who averaged 316 minutes of sleep a night— about 5.2 hours—secreted 50 percent more insulin than their more rested counterparts who averaged 477 minutes of sleep a night, or about 8 hours.

First of all, using the basic tools of the *No-Grain Diet* can help you generate a restful sleep pattern. You can use EFT to address tension, worries, or other discomforts that crop up when you lie down to rest. Regular exercise will prepare your body to relax at bedtime, and here are some additional strategies.

Blissful Sleep Checklist

1. Sleep in complete darkness: Light disrupts the circadian rhythm that governs sleep. If you get up in the middle of the night, keep your bathroom light low or off.

2. No TV before bed: Better yet, get the TV out of the bed-room (or out of the house). Its stimulating effect on the brain will disrupt your sleep cycle.

3. Wear socks to bed: Cold feet may prompt you to awaken in the night.

4. Tune in to your spiritual or religious side: Books, scriptures, prayers, silent meditation, expressions of gratitude, relaxed breathing, sighing and letting go all help you surrender to the blessing of a well-earned rest.

5. Avoid stimulating books: Mystery, adventure, horror, or suspense novels, as well as disturbing news stories, awaken vigilance, and disrupt the calm you are cultivating.

6. No loud alarm clocks: Waking up suddenly is stressful. If you regularly get enough sleep, your body will learn to awaken naturally. I use a dawn simulator that triggers a dimmer switch that gradually turns on the light over forty-five minutes. Almost like a real dawn. I just love it as it is so gentle, and if I need more sleep, I get it without being startled.

7. Journaling: If you lie in bed with your mind racing, keep a journal where you write down your thoughts before bed. Personally, I've done this for fifteen years, but prefer to do it in the morning when my energy is high.

8. Get to bed early: Prior to the widespread use of electricity, people went to bed shortly after sundown, which is nature's way. Most animals do it, too. Our systems, including the adrenals, gallbladder, and liver, dump toxins and recharge between 11 P.M. and 1 A.M. If you're awake, the toxins back up into your entire system, disrupting your health.

9. Keep the temperature at 70 degrees or less: Many people keep their bedrooms too hot. At night, your body cools down and heat makes it harder to enter the normal stages of sleep.

10. Reduce or avoid drugs: Both prescription and over-the-counter medications can affect sleep. In many cases I have found that health conditions can be corrected by natural means. Please consult my website at *www.mercola.com*.

11. Avoid caffeine: An afternoon cup of coffee (or tea) may keep you from falling asleep, as some can't metabolize caffeine efficiently, feeling its effects long after consuming it.

12. Keep electrical devices away from your bed: Keep them at least three feet from the bed to allow your body complete rest.

13. Avoid drinking two hours before bedtime: This reduces the need to arise and go to the bathroom.

14. Take a hot bath, shower, or sauna: When body temperature is raised in the late evening, it will fall at bedtime, facilitating sleep.

15. Remove the clock from view: It will only worry you to stare at it . . . 2 A.M. . . . 3 A.M. . . . 4:30 A.M. . . .

16. Keep your bed for sleeping: If you watch TV or work in bed, you'll find it harder to associate your bed as a place to relax and sleep.

17. If you're menopausal or perimenopausal, get checked out by a good natural medicine physician: Hormonal changes at this time may cause insomnia if not properly addressed.

Melatonin and Its Precursors

The hormone melatonin governs sleep cycles. You can increase your melatonin levels naturally by going out into bright sunlight in the daytime (and by using full-spectrum fluorescent bulbs in the winter). Also helpful is getting absolute darkness at night, using blackout drapes so no light is coming in from the outside.

The amino acids L-tryptophan or 5-hydroxytryptophan (5-HTP) are melatonin precursors, which means they help build your natural melatonin levels. I prefer L-tryptophan, obtained by prescription only. If lifestyle changes and natural supplementation don't work, improve sleep with a melatonin supplement, which you should use only as a last resort, as it's a powerful hormone.

The Basics: Water, Light, and Air

The basic gifts of nature—water, sunlight, rest, movement, healthy foods, and air—are the fuel for life. On this plan, you will learn to connect to these natural sources as our grandparents did, so they can fuel *you*. Then, with optimal energy, you'll be propelled toward your weight-loss and health goals, no longer detoured by unhealthy habits and poor food choices. However, there's one key difference between our times and the past. Unlike our grandparents, we can no longer take such things as a good night's sleep or clean, uncontaminated drinking water for granted. To rediscover the basics, we have to seek nature out, unlearn bad habits, and address and eliminate the harm caused by many substances once thought harmless. Now I'll show you how you can do that.

Water

You Are What You Drink

Most of us don't drink enough water, yet it's one of the most important health steps for any dieter. Dehydration actually prompts you to eat when you really need to *drink,* thus triggering weight gain. It can also cause fatigue, headaches, and constipation. Water makes up more than 70 percent of the body's tissues, supporting nearly every bodily function, from regulating temperature and cushioning joints to bringing oxygen to the cells and removing bodily waste.

Drinking one quart of water for every fifty pounds of body weight is a good starting place, so if you weigh 150 pounds, drink three quarts of water per day, working up to that amount gradually to give your bladder and urinary system time to adjust. Keep a water bottle and sip continually throughout the day since your body only processes one glass per hour.

Water, Water Everywhere

Don't drink tap water! Chlorine (found in nearly all municipal water supplies) is a toxic chemical that should be actively avoided. Given the bacteria, chemicals, and metal traces in many municipal and local water sources, filtering your water is imperative. With different kinds of water and water filtration systems available, here are some basic guidelines for making a choice based on your health and budgetary priorities:

Glass bottled springwater (not drinking water) is a safe but costly choice.

Carbon filters work well to remove particles and bacteria, but don't remove fluoride, which, despite its wide use in preventing tooth decay, can act as a metabolic poison and damage your thyroid. Thyroid impairment is a serious problem affecting millions of women. (In Europe, after much research, they removed fluoride from their water supply.)

Beware of one-gallon cloudy plastic (PVC) containers that transfer dangerous chemicals into the water. Five-gallon containers and clear bottles (polyethylene), made from a better grade of plastic, are better choices.

A Culligan or PUR water filter (sold in most grocery stores) will filter chlorine but not fluoride from your water for just pennies per gallon.

Does your home water supply run through a water softener? If so, divert the softened water away from the kitchen tap into a reverse osmosis system. (See below for more information.)

Avoid distilled water as it has the wrong ionization, pH, polarization, and oxidation potentials, all of which damage your health and drain minerals from your body.

To upgrade your water quality on the Core and Advanced Plans, I recommend that you install a reverse osmosis water filtration system that will remove virtually all contaminants, including fluoride, especially when combined with a pre- and post-carbon filtration system. You can obtain them locally from Home Depot or Coast Filtration (800-542-6723).

. . . And What You Bathe In

To avoid absorbing a large quantity of harmful chlorine from your shower, install a filter on your showerhead. If you take a bath, fill it up from the shower.

. . . And Swim In

Swimming is one of the best exercises on the planet, especially if you swim in the ocean. The balance tips from beneficial to potentially harmful if you swim in a chlorinated pool, where you can absorb a large quantity of chlorine, a toxic substance that can increase your risk of cancer and spontaneous abortions. I strongly advise against it. Alternative pool treatments I recommend are commercial peroxide products like Baquacil, available from pool stores.

Sunlight

For every prescription that's written for heart, diabetes, and weight-loss medications, I'd like to write this one: Take one hour of bright sunlight one time per day—signed, Your Doctor.

Yes, it's true. Getting sunlight produces a cascade of concrete health benefits: First, sun exposure balances your melatonin levels so you sleep better, enjoying the 6.5 hours minimum of sleep needed to regulate your insulin levels.

As well, during summer, one hour of sunshine a day will help stimulate the production of vitamin D, needed for weight loss and countless other healing functions I'll discuss later in this chapter. Exercise caution so that you don't get sunburned, which is the true cause of skin cancer, *not* healthy sun exposure. For optimal sun exposure, please follow basic common sense: go out into the sun at around noontime in the winter, and away from noontime in the summer and in tropical climates, where the sun is hotter. Allow some unfiltered sunlight to hit your retina by not wearing glasses or contacts. Be careful to avoid staring into the sun. You can combine your daily sunbath with a brisk walk.

Full-Spectrum Lighting

If you notice your health symptoms or moods worsen in winter, you can install full-spectrum lighting to compensate for the loss of sun during the winter. But in shopping for them, beware of color-corrected neodymium bulbs. No incandescent light bulb produces a full-spectrum light. Fluorescent lights do, and I recommend either four-foot tubes from Home Depot, or a compact fluorescent full-spectrum bulb that can screw into a standard fixture. Although they are more costly, they produce a bright light on a low wattage, reducing electrical bills and saving you money in the long run.

In the Air

Electromagnetic Fields

Despite their convenience, many common appliances generate electromagnetic fields, harmful to our health, recent studies indicate. Please avoid low-frequency (60 hertz) pulsating electromagnetic fields, found in electric blankets and waterbed heaters. Harmful EMFs are also generated by electric razors and AC/DC plug-in transformers for appliances, as well as car keys with automatic door opening devices.

Smoking: When to Stop

Knowing *when* to quit—smoking, that is—is crucial to successful cessation. That's why I don't recommend quitting when you are just starting this diet. It's too difficult to go off grains and sweets—and tobacco—simultaneously. Once you are solidly into Stabilize on the Core Food Plan, you can quit, and you'll be surprised how easy it is. After all, the tools you've learned and confidence you've built on this diet will be your allies in kicking the butts.

People are often puzzled by this advice since quitting tobacco is generally the first thing most health "experts" ask you to do. Well, what these "experts" do not realize is that sugar is even more dangerous to your health than cigarettes.

That's why it's more important to stop sugar before you stop smoking. If you try to do both at once you will most likely fail to do either. With the energy you'll gain from this diet, quitting smoking will be easier than you expect.

Supplements for Weight Loss and Health

Let's talk about supplements. With the best advice and intentions, some folks have gone a little overboard, taking more supplements than are necessary. I'm convinced we can get most of our nutrients from high-quality food—and that the nutritious diet on all three Food Plans will give you the vast majority of what you need. What's more, the money you save on supplements can be spent on healthier foods.

But due to environmental issues, compounded by the way foods are grown and processed, a few select nutrients cannot be readily supplied by foods—fish oils, vitamin D, and a few others vital to health. Certain select supplements provide key nutrients for total body health and should be taken by everyone. In addition, certain herbs and dietary elements spark weight loss, and you can use them to ignite your metabolism and reverse the insulin cycle. In my practice, I have also found many supplements helpful for specific health conditions, but the ones I'll mention here, anyone can safely use. You'll also find dosages and sources right here in this section of the book.

Listen to Your Body

The single most important guideline for this or any health practice is to listen to your body. When it comes to yourself, you are the ultimate authority. Learn to differentiate between a mild feeling of discomfort which can arise as your body sheds toxins in order to "shift gears" to a higher state of health, and something which just plain doesn't agree with you.

If you find you don't respond well to a food or supplement, respect your body and stop taking it. Your body will always know better than the scientific literature what's good for *you*. Use this God-given instrument to sense the effects of all you do on this program, and you'll experience that your body-mind is your most accurate diagnostic instrument. Tune in emotionally and physically to learn how the program is working for you. Most people notice they feel more energetic, lighter, and healthier in anywhere from a few days to a few weeks.

If not, seek out a knowledgeable health care professional to work *with* you to fine-tune your program. Make sure to pick someone who understands insulin and fat biochemistry. You will find links on my website to recommended practitioners as well. If, for any reason, the Diet is not working for you, make sure that you're using EFT, which I'll discuss fully in the next part of the book.

Supplements to Reduce Cravings

Gymnema Sylvestre

Gymnema is a plant that grows in the tropical forests of central and southern India, where its leaves were chewed to treat diabetes. (It's Hindi name is *gurmar,* which means "destroyer of sugar.") Used for thousands of years by India's Ayurvedic physicians, gymnema has been shown in countless studies to regulate blood sugar levels and glucose metabolism. The dosage is one 500 mg capsule before meals, or as needed to stave off sugar cravings. You can also open the capsule and place the powder on your tongue to eliminate the perception of sugar. It is also available as a gum.

Glutamine

Glutamine, the dominant amino acid in the blood, brain, and cerebrospinal fluid, reduces sugar cravings by suppressing the brain messages that cause them. Dosage ranges between 500 and 1,500 mg before each meal.

Supplements to Boost Your Metabolism

Omega-3 Fats

Omega-3s top my list of essential supplements, and should really be classified as a whole food. Normally, you'd obtain these from fish, but unfortunately most fish is contaminated with mercury and pesticides, as discussed earlier. Fortunately, you *can* get these nutrients from supplements, which have been processed to remove all toxic residues.

Omega-3s speed weight loss by helping the body process fats. As you know, insulin resistance (the major cause of weight gain, diabetes, and a host of other ills) develops in fat tissue, due to impaired fat storage. Consuming omega-3s increases fat processing, thus turning that cycle around.

In addition, omega-3s help reverse and/or prevent:

• Cancer
• Heart disease

- Autoimmune diseases such as MS and rheumatoid arthritis
- Alzheimer's
- Diabetes

What's more, researchers link premature birth, low birth weight, and childhood hyperactivity to low omega-3 levels during pregnancy. So you can see how important omega-3 oils are!

Signs of an Omega-3 Deficiency	
Mental sharpness on awakening	Quality of sleep
Depression/well-being	Memory problems
Weight gain	Dry hair
Brittle fingernails	Dry skin
Allergies	Concentration
Arthritis	Fatigue

Recently, there's been much attention given to all *three* classes of omega oils, 3-6-9. Yet what many don't realize is that most Americans, regularly consuming corn, soy, canola, safflower, and sunflower oils, have an *excess* of dietary omega-6 fats. I recommend that you reduce your omega-6s (by cutting out those so-called healthy oils), while increasing omega-3s by eating omega-3-rich fish oils and flaxseeds. That way you'll have a more health-promoting proportion of these fats stored in your bodily tissues.

I believe the ideal ratio of omega-6 to omega-3 fats is approximately 1:1, but others contend the ideal ratio may be as high as 4:1. Nevertheless, currently the average American has a ratio of 15:1, while many people have dangerous ratios of up to 50:1. Beware of fatty acid supplements that contain omega-6 and omega-9 fats. They will worsen your omega-6 to omega-3 ratio. Avoid them.

Cod Liver Oil Program

Instead, I consider high-quality cod liver oil the best source of omega-3s in the winter, and interestingly, it was *the* all-purpose health remedy back in your grandmother's day. Those from that time who recall its unpleasant taste will feel reassured to know that properly packaged cod liver oil tastes good. Initially, manufacturers did not have the technology to guard against rancidity. Now a number of companies use these tools to supply incredibly fresh and good-tasting oils. I list the best ones on my website, *www.nograindiet*. They taste delicious poured over vegetables or salad. I prefer the liquid to gel caps.

I recommend taking liver oil liquid instead of capsules because the liquid is generally more cost effective. If you are routinely having your vitamin D levels tested, as I recommend, your cod liver oil dosage should be one teaspoon for every 50 pounds of body weight daily. If your vitamin D levels are too high via testing—or if you don't have your vitamin D levels tested at all—your cod liver dosage should be one teaspoon for every 100 pounds of body weight (so one and a half teaspoons for a 150-pound person).

Cod liver oil provides both vitamins A and D. Some authors are concerned about excess vitamin A; however, the amount of vitamin A in one tablespoon of cod liver oil is well under the adult RDA of 10,000 units.

The major concern with cod liver oil is vitamin D toxicity. You can produce vitamin D when you are exposed to sufficient UV from the sun. If you get plenty of sun exposure, please monitor your cod liver oil intake to ensure you don't exceed recommended vitamin D levels. Please review the testing information in my discussion of vitamin D later in this section, as excess vitamin D can produce negative effects, such as osteoporosis and hardening of the arteries.

Along with the cod liver oil, I recommend you take one vitamin E 400-unit supplement per day for its added antioxidant effects, which will protect fats from producing free radicals in your body.

Don't forget the fourth, oft-neglected, oil-soluble vitamin, vitamin K. While you'll get ample amounts with your green vegetable juice, if you are not juicing (or if you have osteoporosis), an extra 1,000 mcg (1 mg) of Vitamin K per day will help ensure increased bone strength.

Cod Liver Oil Protocol

Cod Liver Oil
One teaspoon of liquid for every 50 pounds of body weight for those routinely having their vitamin D levels tested; one

(continued)

> **Cod Liver Oil Protocol** (*continued*)
>
> teaspoon of liquid for every 100 pounds of body weight for those not having their vitamin D levels tested.
> **Vitamin E**
>   400 units, one per day
> **Vitamin K**
>   1,000 mcg (1 mg), one per day

Symptoms of Omega-3 Overdose

The amounts of essential fatty acids you need varies, so fine-tune your dose by following my instructions. After you start the fish oil, if your symptoms improve, continue taking it. However, if after a while your symptoms inexplicably return, stop for a short while to eliminate any residues stored in your system, and then resume with a lower dose.

Unlike your ongoing needs for vitamins and minerals, your essential fatty acid needs are quite variable. If you fine-tune your dose, you can fully benefit from the manifold health benefits that fish oils provide.

Keep Your Oil Fresh

Since fish (and other) oils easily spoil, please refrigerate them after opening. To preserve them, you can use a manual pump, called a "Wine Saver" (purchased from a wine store for $10 to $20) to remove the air from the bottle. Oxygen can damage the highly perishable fats in cod liver oil. The Wine Saver will help you keep it as fresh as possible.

Not Tolerating Fish Oil?

After taking the oil, if you belch, or experience an aftertaste, take cod liver oil next time on an empty stomach. If that doesn't help, your gallbladder may not be emulsifying the fat so you can absorb it, or perhaps your gallbladder has been surgically removed. In either case, taken an enzyme supplement with ample lipase, which helps digest fat. You can also use bile salts to aid digestion.

Other Omega-3 Options

Beyond cod liver oil, another source of omega-3 fat is flax oil, which contains a slightly different form of omega-3—the fatty acid

ALA. Unfortunately, many people (particularly those with insulin resistance) can't convert ALA to the more beneficial EPA and DHA fatty acids. Instead of flax oil, I prefer that you grind up whole flaxseeds (purchased at the health food store) in a food processor or coffee grinder, and then sprinkle them on salads and other foods. Flaxseeds also promote regularity in elimination. If cod liver oil doesn't agree with you, it could be due to the brand you use. Many commercially available oils are oxidized and rancid. Assure you have a high quality product by reviewing the Resource section or *www.nograindiet.com* for our current recommendation of vendors.

Vitamin D

In addition to omega-3 fats, cod liver oil also contains vitamin D, a fat-soluble vitamin found in food. This vitamin helps in the absorption of calcium, to form and maintain strong bones. In addition, adequate D levels aid in weight regulation since this vitamin lowers the secretion of leptin, a hormone produced by fat cells.

Since the 1930s, when rickets (a childhood bone disease) was a widespread U.S health problem, fortified foods, principally milk, have been the main dietary sources of vitamin D.

The healthiest source of vitamin D is produced by your body, which naturally makes the necessary nutrient when your skin is exposed to the sun's ultraviolet rays. These rays vary according to the season, latitude, and time of day, and can be blocked by cloud cover, smog, and sunscreens. For example, in Boston, from November through February, the ultraviolet levels are insufficient to trigger vitamin D synthesis. Sunscreens with a sun protection factor of 8 or more also block the needed UV rays.

As a result, based on your sun exposure and other factors, I recommend that you adjust your vitamin D supplementation to assure you don't take too much of it. If you get regular sun exposure, monitor your 25-hydroxy vitamin D level to check that your range is within 45–55 ng/ml. If it's higher than 40, don't take cod liver oil during the summer months. You can safely start again in the fall if your vitamin D levels are normal. For more details on this test you can go to my website at *http://www.mercola.com/2002/feb/23/vitamin_d_deficiency.htm*. Or just go to *www.mercola.com* or *www.nograindiet.com* and type in vitamin D testing in the search engine query box.

Carnitine

By pumping fat into muscle cells where it's burned as energy rather than stored as fat, carnitine (or L-carnitine) facilitates fat burning, raises energy levels, and reduces cravings, helping you to exercise longer to increase your weight loss. About 80 percent of those who use it see those benefits, while nearly everyone enjoys the boost in energy and well-being. The *No-Grain Diet* enhances carnitine's effectiveness because high insulin levels antagonize carnitine enzymes. To see results, you will need as high a dosage as 1,000 mg of carnitine tartrate, taken three times a day. Take it early in the day, as it is energizing.

Supplements for Total Wellness

Good Bacteria

Nearly everyone can benefit by taking a probiotic to help balance the different strains of bacteria in the intestinal tract. Unless you have a chronic or severe digestive disorder, you probably will only need one or two bottles to normalize your gut flora.

Raw Garlic

To control yeast overgrowth, or candida, in the intestinal tract, I recommend one to three cloves per day. To learn if you have yeast overgrowth, check your tongue in the mirror. A healthy tongue is pink, but if yours is white, this indicates that the rest of your intestinal tract is very likely contaminated. However, if you can't tolerate raw garlic, don't eat it.

Flaxseed

In addition to their health-building omega-3 fats, freshly ground flaxseeds, spread on a salad, or blended into a smoothie, can also initiate bowel regularity just as psyllium products like Metamucil do. However, flax is less expensive, habit forming, and allergenic than psyllium. Flax also contain fibers called lignins, which lower the risk of breast and prostate cancer. You'll find a number of delicious recipes incorporating flax in Chapter Twelve.

Culinary Karma

To Your Health

Whenever you eat while multitasking, or cook by sticking a processed food in a microwave, you'll find you've lost just a few more drops of the joy you used to get from eating and cooking. And that's because *respect* has disappeared from the kitchen. If we respect ourselves, our foods, our meals, our kitchen tools, and the processes used to cook and keep our kitchens clean and healthy, then joy, health, and satisfaction can return to our families, our lives, and our planet. Here are some of my favorite tips for enjoying your food.

Maximize Your Nutrient Intake

Learning how to properly chew your food is an invaluable health technique that's built-in to predigest your food, stimulate the nerves governing digestion, and increase digestive enzyme production. Thoroughly chew your food before swallowing it. Avoid chewing gum, which fools the body, and wastes valuable digestive juices unnecessarily. At mealtime, it's best to avoid talking while chewing, as this interferes with optimal digestion. Drinking fluids with meals dilutes the gastric digestion, making your food more difficult to digest. A few sips of water during the meal is fine.

No Microwaves!

Microwaves seriously deplete foods of their nutrients. Even worse, microwaved food may cause negative changes in your body. It is no surprise that microwave heating of food results in losses of nutrients, because all heating methods do this. However, microwave heating appears to produce the greatest losses. Microwaves are high-frequency electromagnetic waves that alternate in positive and negative directions, causing vibration of food molecules up to 2.5 billion times per second. This creates friction and heat that can destroy the fragile structure of vitamins and enzymes.

Once their structure is altered, they cannot perform their desired function in your body. Clinical studies show that microwave heating of milk or cooking of vegetables is associated with a decline in hemoglobin levels. These reductions may contribute to anemia, rheumatism, fever, and thyroid deficiency.

Keep Your Kitchen and Vegetables Clean

In tests run at Virginia Polytechnic Institute and State University, the following method killed virtually all salmonella, shigella, or E. coli bacteria on heavily contaminated food and surfaces:

To clean vegetables or fruit, spritz them in turn with plain white or apple cider vinegar and 3 percent hydrogen peroxide (available at drugstores). Next rinse them off. Either can be used first, neither is toxic, and you won't get a lingering aftertaste.

These paired sprays can also be used to:

- Sanitize counters, cutting boards, and other kitchen surfaces
- Clean sink drains, refrigerator handles, and faucet handles
- Regularly clean countertops and implements after meat handling
- Disinfect dishcloths and sponges

Now, that you've learned all the fundamentals of the diet and lifestyle changes, in the next part of this book you'll move on to learn how you'll use EFT to stay with the program!

PART 3

OVERCOMING CRAVINGS

CHAPTER 10

EFT: THE BASIC TAPPING MENU (AND HOW TO USE IT)

In the first section of this book, you learned *why* you should follow the *No-Grain Diet*. In the second part, you learned *how* to follow it. Now I want you to get to know your single most powerful tool for *sticking to* the program: the psychological acupressure technique EFT, or Emotional Freedom Technique.

This technique is simple to use. In this chapter, I will first teach you the basic recipe of acupuncture points you'll tap. As you'll discover, it takes about one minute to do the entire sequence. You can learn it in five minutes. To start, I recommend that you read through the next two sections to identify the points on your body. Once you have done that, practice tapping on them in sequence as directed. Then, I'll show you how to use EFT to eliminate cravings and the negative emotions and beliefs underlying them. Having that power will buttress you in staying on the Diet and achieving your weight-loss and health goals.

The EFT Basic Menu

How to Tap

If you've never experienced acupressure before, don't worry. It's easy! For each acupressure point, tap five to seven times, for the duration of one full breath. Since you will use your fingertips to tap on the designated points, to begin please remove your watch, jewelry, long fingernails, or other obstructions to tapping. Numerous acupuncture meridians are located on your fingertips, so make sure to use them, or your finger pads if you have long fingernails.

Originally, EFT Founder Gary Craig taught people to tap by using only the index and middle fingers of one hand. In my version of EFT, I recommend that you use all four fingers of both hands to tap the areas on both sides, allowing you to hit numerous meridian points with every tap.

Tap solidly but gently. Instead of tapping with both hands simultaneously, tap each hand slightly out of phase with the other. This affects the nervous system in a way similar to the alternating eye movement work done in EMDR (Eye Movement Desensitization Rx), a healing modality in wide use for trauma and other psychological disturbances.

While it's ideal to be precise, your tapping will also be effective if you stay *near* the points you'll learn. Each tapping point is below the one before it, going down from the top of your body, making the sequence a snap to memorize. However, you *can* tap the points in any order—just make sure to cover them all.

Where to Tap

Every time you do EFT, tap the following points in order:

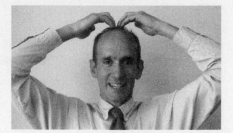

1. TH: top of head along sagittal suture (from front of head to back).

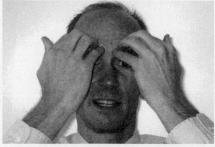

2. EB: along your entire eyebrow, from the outside to the inside area near your nose. (EB for eyebrow.)

3. SE: straight across the bone bordering the outside corner of your eye. Called the zygomatic arch, this is where your eyeglass arm stretches between your eye and ear. (SE for side of the eye.)

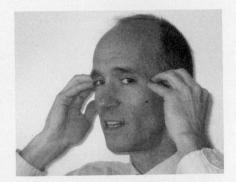

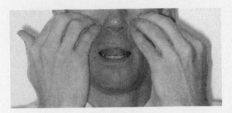

4. UE: the area under both eyes as close as possible to your eye without touching it. (UE for under the eye.)

5. UN: between the bottom of your nose and the top of your upper lip. (UN for under the nose.)

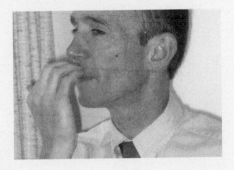

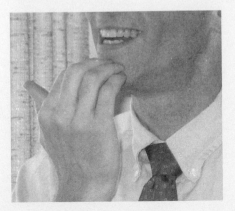

6. Ch: midway between your lower lip and the point of your chin. (Ch for chin.)

7. CB: the junction where your sternum (breastbone), collarbone, and first rib meet. (CB for collarbone, even though it's not on the collarbone.) To locate this point, first place your forefinger on the U-shaped notch at the top of the breastbone (about where a man would knot his tie). From there, move your forefinger down toward the navel one inch and then go to the left (or right) one inch. Acupuncturists call this point Kidney 27.

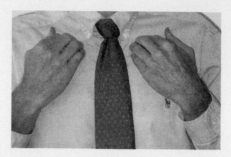

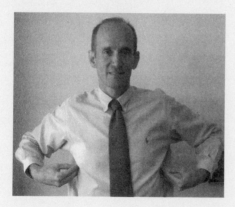

8. UA: on the side of the body, four inches below the armpit, at a point even with the nipple (for men) or in the middle of the bra strap (for women). (UA for under the arm.)

9. and 10. The last points are the insides of each wrist, which you will tap in turn.

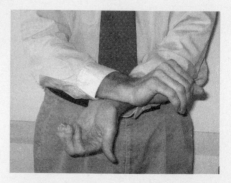

To learn more about EFT, I encourage you to go on-line to *www.mercola.com* to download my EFT Manual, or go to Gary Craig's website, *www.emofree.com*, where you can download his EFT Manual and sign up to receive his free newsletter.

Creating your Healing Phrase

What to Say While You Tap

As you learned in Chapter Four, EFT works by *deleting* undesirable cravings and feelings from your mind and body's memory. You will need to first *identify* the craving, emotion, sensation, or belief that you want to eliminate. Then to focus your attention on it, you will need to craft a phrase that captures the essence of what you want to remove. You will say this phrase out loud, or if you're in public, you may want to say it quietly, or even just silently concentrate on it. Sometimes homing in on that phrase takes a little work, and I'll provide further tips on how to do that in the next chapter.

But for now, let's say that you want to eliminate a craving for chocolate cake. You decide to use the phrase "I crave this piece of chocolate fudge cake." You would then combine *your* phrase with the traditional EFT "Setup," which is the following:

"Even though _____, I deeply and completely accept myself."

This makes *your* healing statement:

"Even though *I crave this piece of chocolate fudge cake,* I deeply and completely accept myself."

Here are some additional examples:

"Even though *I want to eat the entire dozen doughnuts,* I deeply and completely accept myself."

"Even though *I want to have pizza,* I deeply and completely accept myself."

"Even though *I'm sure to be tempted by the kids' candy on Halloween,* I deeply and completely accept myself."

Remember, whatever the problem, the blank is always filled in with a brief description of what you want to address.

Fine-Tuning the Setup

As you start, make sure that the Setup phrase you regularly use rings true for you. While I prefer the basic Setup, which has a good track record, if needed you can also vary it, as long as you follow the basic format: first acknowledge the problem, then create self-acceptance despite it.

Beyond the basic model, here are some other good choices:

"Even though _____, I deeply love and accept myself."

"I accept myself even though I have this _____."

"Even though I have this _____, I deeply and profoundly accept myself."

"I love and accept myself even though I have this _____."

"Even though _____, I'm okay."

"Although I have this _____, I'm a worthwhile person."

The Reminder Phrase

Sometimes, it will take more than one round of tapping to eliminate your craving or issue. If so, on subsequent rounds, you can shorten the formula by instead using a "reminder phrase." This is equally effective, freeing you from repeating the entire lengthy formula each time.

As your reminder, use your key phrase (or a portion of it), as in:

"Even though *I have this craving for chocolate ice cream,* I deeply and completely accept myself." *Reminder phrase:* "chocolate ice cream."

"Even though *I feel lousy today,* I deeply and completely accept myself." *Reminder phrase:* "feeling lousy."

In other words, after the first round, tap on your reminder phrase "chocolate ice cream" or "feeling lousy" all by itself.

People often ask me what to do in situations where they need to do EFT in a public place. Suppose you're kicking your coffee habit. You find yourself on a busy street, passing Starbucks. You're feeling a strong craving for a mocha latte and cookie, but you don't want to stand out in the crowd by tapping and saying your statement. What should you do? Don't worry. After some private practice, you can use only two fingers of one hand and say the statements silently or softly under your breath. This way you can always use EFT inconspicuously whenever you need it.

Undoing Cravings from the Source

Now that you know the basics of how to use EFT, you are ready to incorporate this highly effective technique into your weight-loss program. The three keys to success with EFT are:

- Starting to use it
- Using it regularly
- Fine-tuning your skills to use it for every issue blocking your health and weight-loss goals

Cravings That Prompt You to Eat

Use EFT when you experience a craving for grains, starches, and sweets, or whenever you feel a craving for a food not on this plan. For example, if you suddenly feel the urge to go into the kitchen and eat a candy bar, use EFT right there and then. On the other hand, perhaps you know you'll be dining tomorrow evening with friends at a restaurant with delicious bread and desserts. Or your family will visit Aunt Margaret next weekend and she makes a really knockout strawberry rhubarb pie. Be vigilant: once you notice that you are picturing the pie and imagining yourself eating it, take that as a warning. Use EFT right away to rid yourself of the craving *in advance*. You can also use EFT to imagine yourself passing on the pie, but we'll explore more thoroughly how to input new information into your body-mind in the next chapter.

In addition to sudden cravings and future challenges, there may be regular food patterns you need to change to stay on the *No-Grain Diet*. Perhaps you are in the habit of eating a bagel every morning at work. If so, you would need to choose a healthier snack, and also tap away your bagel craving. Maybe you always eat popcorn at the movies. You need to bring a healthier snack, and tap away your popcorn habit. Or if late night eating or binge eating is a problem for you, you may need regular EFT to end those habits.

You may have to tap whenever you experience cravings, watching them gradually lessen and then disappear over time. You can repeat your chosen formulation as often as ten to twenty times per day for as long as five days. If the craving or problem persists even after this amount of time, probe more deeply to uncover hidden blocks in your emotions, beliefs, or energy system. Throughout this and the next chapter, I'll show you how to do that.

Quite often, you'll find that a food craving comes bundled with other feelings you also must address to successfully eliminate it. When this occurs, patiently unravel the bundle strand by strand so that you can focus one by one on each of the contributing factors, and tap it away. For example, if your family regularly has a special French toast brunch every Sunday, you may need to do three things:

- Change the menu (at least for yourself)
- Address the craving for the eliminated food
- Deal with the feelings that accompany this change

By now it's already clear to you that you would address the craving by tapping on "Even though *I want to eat that French toast,* I deeply and completely accept myself."

But that alone may not be successful because of the other feelings involved. Not joining in with the rest of your family at this special meal could make you feel alone, deprived, or perhaps, overworked since you now must prepare two different dishes. This experience might be connected to other negative feelings, experiences, beliefs, or memories, such as "I'm always on the outside looking in," or "Everyone else gets to enjoy themselves," or "I have to do everything." Any of those associated feelings might sabotage you until you address them. If a craving persists beyond one week, assume that you need to probe further to identify and eliminate the emotional strand.

Emotions That Prompt You to Eat

It's easy to recognize immediate cravings for particular foods, or the hunger that drives you into a fast-food outlet, bakery, or pizzeria. But it's equally important for you to learn to notice *emotions* that prompt you to eat. Sometimes, the emotion is obvious, as in these examples:

"Even though *I'm depressed and really deserve that bagel,* I deeply and completely accept myself."

"Even though *I'm angry at my boyfriend and want to comfort myself with a hot chocolate,* I deeply and completely accept myself."

But sometimes, the connection between your craving and its emotional source may be less obvious.

> At an EFT demonstration before four hundred clinical nutritionists, Jennifer, a physician, had a very strong craving for Rice Krispies treats offered in the exhibit area. After one round of tapping, her eyes filled with tears and she began to weep. Jennifer recalled that, when she was a small child and reached out to her mother, her mother instead used to give her M&M treats to get her out of her hair.
>
> Jennifer's craving for the treats was only the superficial problem. The real issue was her craving for the love and attention that her mother could not provide, offering instead the inferior candy substitute. After she tapped on "even though I craved my mom's attention," Jennifer's cravings for sweets disappeared, never to return.

Just like Jennifer, you have your own personal reasons for craving unhealthy foods, and on the *No-Grain Diet,* you'll discover precisely what those are. For some people, self-awareness is valuable for its own sake, yet many people feel that if there's nothing to do about painful things, why bother bringing them up? Let me reassure you: now it's safer than ever before to dig a little deeper, to the roots of your eating problem, because whatever you uncover, you can handle it—with EFT. EFT bridges the gap between your emotions and your actions, erasing the disconnection between your desire for weight loss and your actual behavior. For many, this is the missing link in permanent weight loss. In the next chapter, I'll show you more about how to home in on the emotions that stimulate you to eat, and to craft your healing phrases based on what you find.

But first, review my Emotional Survey, which covers some of the common wants, lacks, and feelings that prompt many people to eat, and note if any of them motivate you.

Emotional Survey

Do I want?
- Love
- Sex
- Security
- Support

- Reassurance
- Friendship
- Comfort
- Communication

Do I lack?
- Confidence
- Self-esteem
- Contentment

- Job satisfaction
- Satisfying relationship

Do I feel?
- Sad or grief-stricken
- Lonely
- Depressed
- Irritated
- Angry or frustrated
- Annoyed
- Hurt

- A loss
- Abandoned
- Overwhelmed
- Worried
- Agitated
- Anxious

You can always check back to the Emotional Survey to help identify your emotional prompts. Often, in simply reviewing the survey questions, the real reason will suddenly occur to you. If that happens, jot it down so you can work with it.

Hidden Beliefs

If you're like most people, you're probably aware of some of your basic beliefs, which may include common ones like "It's a free country," or "If you work hard, you'll succeed," or "I want what's best for my children." But below your *conscious* beliefs are *hidden* beliefs that influence your actions, without your realizing it. Sometimes, these even contradict your conscious beliefs. For example, if your dad was very critical of you, in addition to your conscious belief "If you work hard, you'll succeed," you'll also carry the hidden belief "I can never get it right." As a result, you'll probably act in a way that fulfills *both* beliefs. You'll work hard, and you won't get it right!

And guess what: those conflicting beliefs will influence you in your job, relationships, and yes, even in your weight-loss program. Why? Because *your body will always work to fulfill your beliefs,* both conscious and hidden. The life experience you create for yourself is built within the parameters of your beliefs. Think of beliefs as a fence that surrounds and contains your life territory. If your beliefs are very constricting, your freedom of action will be quite limited. However, you can expand that territory by using EFT.

You formed your conscious beliefs based upon what you heard in your home, school, work, or religious group. But you formed hidden beliefs based on what important others communicated, and also from what you saw and experienced. To go back to the above example, your father may have actively criticized you when you helped out with chores, reenforcing the perception "I can't get it right." Or perhaps *his* business failed, leading you to believe that success was impossible. In either case, your belief is a roadblock to success in any undertaking. Hidden beliefs can afflict your self-esteem, empowerment, and effectiveness, thus contributing *indirectly* to your weight gain. That's why it's important to identify and eliminate them.

Uncovering beliefs may require some digging. Sometimes, as you tap, a memory, image, person, place, or event may suddenly come to mind. Pay attention to what comes up, as it may reveal clues that will help you to uncover your blockages. Also listen carefully to inner voices, messages, or dictates. Often these lead toward beliefs that hold you back, beliefs that have undermined your previous weight-loss attempts. Once you are able to identify them and use them in an EFT tapping round, their power over you will dissipate.

Whenever you notice that your internal self-talk includes self-critical thoughts, painful images, or uncomfortable feelings, you can free yourself by simply loving and accepting yourself while tapping on your acupuncture meridians. Listen to concerns swirling in your mind, and see if you can trace them back to their source.

Here are some examples:

Your concern: I'm sure I won't be able to do this diet.
Your reason: Dad always called me a failure.
Your belief: "I'm a failure at everything."
Your healing statement: "Even though *I believe that I'm a failure at everything and will surely fail on this diet,* I deeply and completely accept myself."

Your concern: I'm worried weight loss might threaten my marriage.
Your reason: Our whole family was scandalized when Cousin Betty had an affair after she became slim.
Your belief: "Losing weight will inevitably cause me to behave immorally."
Your healing statement: "Even though *I'm afraid to lose weight because I believe I will act like Cousin Betty,* I deeply and completely accept myself."

Your concern: Like all of my sisters and cousins, I'll never lose weight.
Your reason: Mom said that we're all overweight because it's in our genes.
Your belief: "I am biologically determined to be fat and there's nothing I can do about it."
Your healing statement: "Even though *I believe it's physically impossible for me to lose weight,* I deeply and completely accept myself."

Perhaps as you read this you feel a sense of skepticism. Or you may notice that you're having difficulty uncovering or eliminating beliefs. If so, it's quite possible that you hold the common belief that "These are my beliefs and there's nothing I can do about them." That's natural if you've never felt a belief dissolving and a new opportunity to experience life opening before you. If that's the case for you, I want you to tap on the following: "Even though *I believe that I can't change my beliefs,* I deeply and completely accept myself."

Yes, your beliefs can change. Using EFT, you can change them and move on to a slimmer, healthier you.

Social Eating

While we all eat for nourishment and enjoyment, eating is also a social activity. That's why altering your diet may affect your interactions with others. If up until now you and another mom from your toddlers' play group regularly took the kids out for ice cream and gossip, how can you keep up that fun relationship, while staying on the Diet? Or suppose that to meet a deadline at work, your department is in the habit of ordering in sandwiches. Now you can't eat them. What will you do? Every summer, you and your mate join another family for a Beach Weekend, where beer, hot dogs, corn on the cob, and steamed clams are usually eaten. You hate to become a nuisance by changing a traditional celebration that others enjoy.

Every problem has a solution. Don't let social pressures knock you off your weight-loss program. I want you to be prepared to deal with social eating whenever it arises. The best way to do that is to think ahead and plan. For example, instead of going for ice cream, maybe, if asked, your friend would like to join you for a mom and toddler yoga class. If the office is ordering sandwiches, you could order a salad. Or you could plan to bring in a salad and eat it with the turkey (minus the bread) taken from a turkey sandwich. In place of the usual foods at your summer weekend, you could make plans to prepare the delicious coleslaw recipe in Chapter Twelve and barbecued steaks and chicken. Or you could suggest that you and your friends plan to visit a different city and attend its museums, concerts, or theater. You could suggest that you take a health-oriented culinary workshop together, or visit a spa where healthy food is emphasized.

Be creative. Use the following Social Eating Checklist to troubleshoot situations where going along with others can endanger your diet.

Social Eating Checklist

Daily Life
- Breakfast at home or office
- Snacks or coffee breaks
- Business lunches
- Social lunches
- Meals or informal get-togethers with friends
- Activities with kids, teens, and their friends
- Afternoon teas and snacks
- Family, romantic, business, school, or social dinners
- Regular recreational activities
- Community, volunteer, or religious group activities
- Social drinking
- Professional meetings, conferences, and workshops

Leisure Activities
- Social gatherings
- Family visits
- Sports activities
- Watching television
- Movies
- Brunches, parties, social dinners, cocktail parties
- Worship, potlucks, and religious group events
- Travel
- Shopping
- Cultural events

Seasonal Activities and Celebrations
- July 4th picnic or beach gatherings
- Holiday celebrations
- Weddings, celebrations, birthday parties, and showers
- Family gatherings and ethnic events
- Halloween, Thanksgiving, and other celebrations oriented around traditional meals and foods

Sometimes the hardest thing is just saying "No." If you do what's best for your own well-being, your friends, loved ones, coworkers, and family will be supportive if they care for you. In most cases, they probably won't even notice. But if anyone gives you a hard time, don't let it throw you. First, use EFT to tap away the anxiety or concern sparked by their disapproval. Next, consider where they're coming from. Perhaps that person needs to lose a few pounds. Perhaps they are threatened because they fear losing you, or are envious. Reassuring them of your love or friendship will help in many cases. If not, you will need to take active steps to deal with your feelings about their behavior, and to let them know that your weight and health are your concern.

But whatever their problem is, remember it's theirs, not yours. Keep your perspective and keep on tapping away any distress.

Adjusting to Weight Loss

Looking ahead to your future weight loss, let's consider the reasons why many yo-yo on diets, losing weight only to gain it back. I don't want that to happen to you. To avoid this common fate, let's look at why it occurs. Slimming down is something you've hoped for and worked hard to achieve. Yet, as you shed those excess pounds, you simultaneously shed your old self-image, or certain aspects of it. Instead of being a victim of your addictions, you are empowered. Instead of succumbing to painful emotions, you have addressed them and moved on. Your options have expanded; your self-esteem has been boosted. Adjusting to even positive changes can be challenging, especially when the weight loss is dramatic. That's why it's essential to be prepared for the challenges of transition and use EFT to deal with them.

Weight-Loss Adjustment Checklist

- Needing new clothes
- Being able to wear different kind of styles, colors, and hairdos
- Reactions from loved ones, friends, colleagues, and family members

(continued)

Weight-Loss Adjustment Checklist (*continued*)

- Strangers and acquaintances respond to you differently
- The opposite sex may be more attracted to you
- Overweight people no longer recognize you as one of them
- Able to participate in sports and other new leisuretime activities
- More vitality and energy
- Less willing to accept unfavorable life circumstances
- Noticing things you feel more profoundly
- Responding to life challenges and occurrences in new ways
- Renewed sense of self-worth
- Drawn to new life goals

Look through this checklist and note any that might trigger you to eat unwisely. First of all, recognize that it's natural to feel overwhelmed. But now, with EFT, you can take active steps to handle your "overwhelm" so that it doesn't undo all your efforts.

For example, you can use EFT to address emotions or fears like "I'm afraid people will stare at me if I wear a two-piece to the community pool." Or perhaps, with your new sense of self-worth, you no longer want to accept a "glass ceiling" at work. Whatever the situation, EFT is a resource.

Delving into Emotional Blocks to Weight Loss

After you have addressed one facet of an issue, another will often emerge. Or you may find that a craving doesn't subside until you deal with the emotion with which it's intertwined. Be persistent, and monitor your progress. Above all, don't judge yourself for your feelings or beliefs. Acknowledge them, love yourself, and allow them to pass. If they seem strange, don't be concerned. Be a neutral observer.

A sixty-four-year-old grandmother had difficulty losing weight. As she tapped her first round of EFT, she suddenly recalled that she was last at her normal weight during a pregnancy thirty years earlier. Even though her conscious mind recognized that, at age sixty-four, she could not become pregnant, her subconscious held the belief that if she achieved her goal weight, she would do just that. Normal weight and pregnancy were intertwined and stored together in her body's sense memory.

Fortunately, EFT unlocked this long held association. After she completed tapping, she was able to lose the twenty-two pounds that she had carried for over thirty years.

This woman's experience reveals how tenaciously the body-mind holds an experience, belief, or emotion, whether or not it's healthy, or even makes sense! But the good news is that EFT will help your body-mind disengage from non-optimal internal programming, experiences, memories, and beliefs. But that's not all! You can also use EFT to actively *program* your system with positive beliefs, emotions, and attitudes that are aligned with your goals and dreams.

Up until today, if you're like most of the people I see in my office, you may not have realized that all the things you say, actively do, or quietly think are actually programming you, your experience, and your future. You have the power to take control of that with EFT. In the next chapter, I'll share with you how to probe for underlying emotions and beliefs that block your weight-loss progress, along with some advanced skills in using EFT.

CHAPTER 11

EFT: REALLY GETTING IT!

E FT is integral to the *No-Grain Diet*. It's the special ingredient that empowers you to stay on the diet until you've achieved your goals. Although thousands around the world have attained astounding results with EFT, I know that it's probably new to you, so in this chapter I'll troubleshoot every possible obstacle to your gaining complete ease with it.

First, I'll get you started. Next, you'll learn to use a process to uncover the issues that underlie your weight gain. Then, you'll find out about a new way to use affirmations to troubleshoot hidden obstacles. Finally, you'll learn to install *positive* affirmations more powerfully by combining them with EFT. Use the exercises in this chapter as you would a workbook. Get out your notebook. Immerse yourself in these new tools for permanent weight loss. Let's start!

Your EFT practice should feel natural and comfortable, tailor-made to your needs, issues, and goals. Please **don't ever worry about doing EFT wrong. You can't!**

EFT is flexible. You can change the Setup, fine-tune your healing phrase, tap at any strength, in any order, miss a few points, and it will still work for you—as long as you tune in to the problem you want to erase and do it!

Take the time to check out the sites on the web listed in the Resources section of this book. There you'll see the countless effective ways to do EFT and also explore the wide variety of related energy and psychological acupressure techniques. Once you see the great variety of ways people use EFT, you'll realize that doing it perfectly matters less than doing it. Period.

If you feel comfortable using EFT, please skip ahead to page 186, where you'll find exercises to help you prospect for undermining emotions and beliefs. But if you've had trouble getting started, please read on to get over that initial hump.

Obstacles to Doing It!

In my work with people, I've come across every kind of blockage in getting started with this powerful and effective tool. Here are three of the most common:

I forgot about it!

"Forgetting" is one of the most frequent excuses. For example, my patient Angela had skipped over the EFT exercises, since she thought tapping sounded "silly." Initially, she followed the diet well without that added support. Then came her cousin's wedding, where Angie broke her diet with a generous portion of wedding cake, followed by a full week of indulging in sweets once she returned home.

Irresistible EFT

Another patient of mine, Jerome, was an ex-smoker. While quitting, he got into the habit of sucking on sourball candies. At the outset of his diet, Jerome used EFT and felt no candy craving for four days. Formerly, he'd eaten a sourball every waking hour. On the fifth day, Jerome craved a candy, which led to another. Jerome returned to his habit. Though EFT had worked just fine, Jerome was taken off-guard when he felt a craving. At that critical moment, he "didn't bother" to use it because it "somehow seemed too simple," Jerome said.

What Angela and Jerome experienced is quite common. As you know from the previous chapter, EFT can eliminate subtle, undermining beliefs, like Angela's ("silly") or Jerome's ("too simple"). But what if a belief blocks you from using EFT, causing you to "forget" EFT or dismiss it? Psychologists call this *resistance*. Perhaps at some time you've felt your body-mind rebel or shut down in the face of something you know is beneficial. You want to do it but you can't. In EFT, we view this problem as an energetic misalignment, called "psychological reversal," which causes your body-mind to work against you. Fortunately, you can *use EFT* to address even the *resistance to doing EFT*.

My Problem Left . . . Somehow

Here's another common experience: after a round or two of EFT, you *forget the problem itself* and no longer feel bothered by it. My patient Sylvia felt deeply hurt by her sister-in-law's putdown, and launched into a round of binge eating. She successfully used EFT to call a halt to this downward spiral. Before tapping, she couldn't get Rita's harsh words out of her mind; afterward *she couldn't recall them.* The whole incident lost its charge, and faded. Once Sylvia could no longer remember her problem, she forgot that EFT helped, so that the next time she faced a craving, it didn't occur to her to call upon EFT.

I've seen literally scores of people attribute their problem's sudden disappearance to confusion caused by all that tapping. But they're mistaken. Here's what's really going on: as EFT removes the painful thought, feeling, or experience, it reorganizes your energy and nervous system. As you adjust to this new way of being, you feel different, and that's why people sometimes mistake the change for confusion.

Breaking Through

The mechanics of EFT are easy to master. Crafting your healing phrases you'll perfect over time. But if you've had trouble getting started, read through the following statements, designed to address and eliminate all forms of reversal. Select one to use or modify right now.

Troubleshooting:

The problem: Feeling uncomfortable or resisting doing EFT.
The solution: Tapping on your choice of the following EFT
    phrases: "Even though I (*choose one*):
tried EFT and didn't do it right,
am not sure I know how to do EFT correctly,
am not sure I need to do EFT,
am not sure I will use EFT again,
am unclear why EFT works,
feel a little strange doing EFT,
wish EFT would help but am afraid it won't,
I deeply and completely accept myself."

OR:

"Even though I feel too (*choose one*):
inadequate, busy, preoccupied,
unworthy, fat, incompetent,
lazy, unfortunate, stressed,
to do EFT successfully, I deeply and completely accept myself."

OR:

"Even though I believe that EFT is (*choose one*):
unscientific, silly, ridiculous,
hocus pocus, a waste of time,
boring, too easy to work,
too far out, hard to do right,
difficult to understand,
overly complicated, confusing,
easy to forget, embarrassing to do in public,
I deeply and completely accept myself."

If you don't recognize a phrase that rings true for you, please
write one down in the space provided here.

"Even though _____, I deeply and completely accept myself."

Congratulations! You've just done EFT. Now that you're familiar with the basic tapping sequence, you can move on to garner EFT's full benefits.

Global Barriers to Weight Loss

Honoring What Comes Up

People use "bad" foods to avoid "bad" feelings. Generous portions, comfort foods, sweets, treats, and snacks help stuff down feelings that don't feel good. While no feelings are truly bad, if you eat because you are feeling sad, angry, frustrated, helpless, or unworthy, then you are using food not for health but to cover your emotions. Somewhere along the line you learned that it was better to eat than to allow yourself to feel, and act on your feelings.

If you suddenly stop eating this way—guess what happens? All those "bad" feelings come up. If you attempt to diet without preparing for this natural reaction, it will be near impossible to maintain your weight loss. You will succeed only if you learn how to accept your emotions. Use EFT to increase your comfort in experiencing them.

On the Diet, this process of discovery will unfold naturally, with new information about what imprisons you in weight gain emerging over time. As with the child's toy the Magic Eight-Ball, messages float up from the depths within to reveal themselves. You never know what's going to come up next.

Cultivate an attitude of curiosity about what emerges, along with faith about the outcome. Work with yourself gently. Fundamental to successful weight loss is getting to know and make friends with yourself and with your body. Beating yourself up is not the way to go. Instead, at all times, treat your own issues, feelings, and experiences—and your past, present, and future self—with love and respect.

Your mind-body is wondrous: a subtle complex of life force, energy, feeling, thought, structure, and biochemistry. All levels of your being are interrelated. From this vast inner archive, you can learn to access valuable information about yourself to activate your weight-loss and healing process. Honor what comes up and proceed at your own pace and comfort level.

Eliminate Threats to Weight Loss

People often ask, "Is it really necessary to delve into my emotions and beliefs?" The answer is "Yes and no."

It's not necessary if you find that tapping on cravings works, as it does for many people. But if you find blocks between you and dietary success than the answer is a resounding "Yes!" If your cravings and bad eating habits persist, if you've reached a plateau, if you feel unmotivated, unworthy, or lack confidence that you can continue on the Diet and achieve your weight-loss goals, than it's best to address these underlying emotional patterns and beliefs.

EFT can help you undo the issues that created the overweight you, *if* you know what they are. To help open that inner archive of vital information, I'd like to introduce you to two powerful techniques.

Four Steps to Eternal Slimness

The first process contains four steps that can be applied to anything blocking your weight-loss efforts. Whether it's an eating habit, feeling, belief, social eating challenge, or self-image issue, use the four steps. At first, you may not even know the nature of your obstacle, and that's okay. Following the process will reveal it.

The Four Steps

1. First, notice and write down your challenge (which may be a feeling, belief, memory, experience, doubt, concern, or emotion, directed toward self or others).

2. Second, ask yourself *Why? Why* this challenge? Once you are clear, you are ready to . . .

3. Brainstorm a strategy to address the challenge, and

4. Develop a healing phrase to use with EFT.

Here's how to use the process to troubleshoot undesirable eating habits. Address them in advance, so that they don't come up and catch you off guard. *Prepare* to deal with them, so that you remain in control, on course, and on the diet. You *can* succeed and you *will* succeed through this process.

Please consult the Daily Eating Pattern Checklist below. Note all meals and times of day where you crave unhealthy foods, or indulge in unhealthy eating patterns. Ultimately, for each noted item, you will do all four steps, but right now, I want you to pick just *one* pattern or challenge to follow through the four steps so that you get the hang of it.

Daily Eating Pattern Checklist

Breakfast
Coffee break
Midmorning snack
Lunch
Afternoon snack
End of day/home from work snacking
Cocktail hour
Dinner
Bedtime snack
Late night eating

Follow the Four Steps

Step One: Write down the time, the occasion, your food challenge or issue, and *why* it makes you feel vulnerable to eating unhealthy foods.

For example, my patient, Claire had the tendency to awaken in the middle of the night for milk and cookies. In her notebook, she wrote, "Late night, unable to sleep, eating milk and cookies to calm myself."

Step Two: Ask yourself *why*. To do this, read over what you've written, and develop at least one more why question. Make it a deeper why.

In Claire's case, she asked two questions: "Why can't I sleep through the night?" and "Why do cookies calm me down?"

To answer the first question, Claire consulted my Blissful Sleep Checklist (on page 147 of Chapter Nine) and recognized that her regular habit of television viewing before bed was a blissful sleep no-no.

In mulling over the second question, Claire realized that eating milk and cookies reminded her of when she was a little girl. On his rare visits following her parents' divorce, her dad would take her over to his mom's home for milk and cookies. She associated this treat with the father whose presence she missed.

Claire's probing helped her to get to the bottom of her issue through asking why.

Find the Deeper Why

Whenever you ask yourself *why,* there are many levels of reasons. Responses like "I just felt like it . . ." or "That's what I've always done . . ." or "It's no different from what everyone else does . . ." function like dead-ends, opening no further pathway to healing or understanding. If instead you find arising within you a deep feeling, memory, insight, bodily sensation, or understanding, know that you have accessed the *deeper why.* Always aim for the deeper why. If, at first, you don't reach it, relax, and try again.

Troubleshooting

The problem: If you're stuck with a dead-end why, and can't go further, you may be in a state of resistance or psychological reversal. To go forward, first address this state.
The solution: Use EFT to tap on phrases to address it.
Suggested phrases: "Even though (*choose one or modify as you wish*) *I don't know why, I haven't a clue why, I feel confused about why, I could care less why, I can't reveal to myself why, my body refuses to divulge why, it's not safe for me to know why . . .*"

Step Three: Brainstorm a strategy to address the challenge: Now that you know the problem, figure out a way to solve it.

Claire's strategy for addressing her insomnia was to cut out late night TV viewing.

Her strategy for the second issue was to use EFT to disconnect the linkage between her current cookie habit and her past experience of missing her father.

Step Four: Develop a healing phrase for use with EFT.

Claire came up with "Even though I eat cookies and milk because I missed my daddy, I deeply love and accept myself."

Troubleshooting:

The problem: You can't come up with a strategy.
The solution: Tap on "Even though I can't devise a strategy . . ."
The problem: You have trouble following through on a strategy.
The solution: Tap on "Even though I lack the motivation to follow through on my plan to _____ . . ." or "Even though I feel as though I'll never get over (my eating habit) by (using this strategy) . . ."

EFT Comes Alive

As Claire and many others have found, developing your awareness, creating strategies, and using EFT makes a powerful combination for overcoming cravings and unhealthy eating habits. Don't worry if it takes a few tries until you hit upon the right phrase to use with your EFT Setup. Make sure the phrase rings true for you. Speak in your own voice. If your linked emotion first occurred in childhood, choose words that speak to the child in you. For example, don't say, "my father," say "Daddy" or "Pops," or whatever you called him.

Simplify your phrase so that it's easy to say, and you'll attain the same results. For example, through the four-step process, my patient

Edith discovered that her daily chocolate habit stemmed from a childhood incident. In her notebook, Edith first captured it as "Even though I felt abandoned that day my parents lost me at the circus, and only found comfort later when Grandma gave me chocolate, so that I now crave chocolate every day . . ."

When Edith tried to tap on that phrase, she found it too long to remember and pronounce, so she streamlined it to "Even though I eat chocolate to feel less abandoned as I did that time at the circus . . ." While saying this easier phrase, Edith simultaneously created a mental image of that evening, including all that she saw, heard, smelled, and felt. She pictured the Ferris wheel, smelled the cotton candy, heard the hawker's cry, felt her anxiety about finding her parents, and recalled the chill of the evening air. Let all your senses work for you as Edith did. Imagining the situation as vividly as possible gives your nervous system a three-dimensional replay of the real event—with a new outcome, created by you. In that new outcome, instead of feeling unloved and alone, you will feel loved and empowered because love and acceptance are built right into the Setup. You are not denying the reality of what occurred, you are incorporating that reality into your life experience in a way that no longer harms you. To simplify further, you could also say, "chocolate—circus," which would suffice to conjure up the whole incident for you.

Applying the Four Steps to Other Issues

Use the process you've just learned for any kind of obstacle or challenge you encounter on your path to weight loss, including:

1. Overcoming internal barriers to weight loss
2. Eliminating cravings permanently
3. Releasing underlying emotions causing you to eat and gain weight
4. Addressing hidden beliefs that undermine your weight loss
5. Staying steadfast in the face of social challenges that threaten your diet

6. Shifting self-image and body image to support your emergence into the new you

7. Remaining slim and addiction-free forever

Use it to identify potential cravings, and future social eating challenges. Use it to uncover emotions, beliefs, and self-image deficits that bar your way. Consult the Emotional Survey (on page 174), the Social Eating Checklist (on page 178), the Weight-Loss Adjustment Checklist and/or the Self-Image Survey (on page 179) to help you surface hidden issues to work with.

Finally, if accessing your feelings and concerns is new, and you need help getting started, additional support is available. Throughout the U.S. and abroad, there are many able practitioners trained in using EFT. To find one near you, please consult the listings in the Resources section of this book (which will be updated on my website). Assistance with EFT doesn't have to be costly or lengthy. Often, with a little boost at the start, you can quickly go on to use EFT independently.

The Power of Affirmations

You may already be familiar with affirmations, used as a tool to actively nourish your entire being with optimal beliefs and goals. Personally, I am a great believer in using them to program your mind. I know from personal experience that one can derive great benefit from nourishing oneself daily with self-acceptance, positive thoughts, and intentions. I highly recommend doing them before bedtime to program your unconscious mind as you sleep. Starting the day with affirmations is also very helpful. If telling yourself what you intend or believe seems unusual, just remember this: your mind is generating thoughts and beliefs all the time. If they are critical or negative, they affect you, even if you are not clearly aware of them. So why not make them positive and beneficial?

In formulating an affirmation, remember these simple guidelines:

1. Always state your goal positively, for example, "I am slim . . ." or "I choose to be slim . . ." instead of "I am no longer fat . . . ."

2. Always formulate your intention *in the present tense* to avoid unwittingly making your goal out of reach, as in "I *am* slim and strong . . ." rather than "I *will be* slim and strong . . ."

Some resist affirmations because "it's untrue to say I'm slim when I'm forty pounds overweight." That's why EFT founder Gary Craig likes to use affirmations in an entirely different way: to surface unconscious beliefs. In his technique, you speak your affirmation, and then wait for what Gary calls a "tail-ender," a belief that tags along with your affirmation and negates it. For example, Cindy decided to use the affirmation "I'm svelte and gorgeous." After she said it, she listened carefully and inside her mind heard, "No, you're not, you're a fat pig and always will be." This was the familiar harsh voice of a punitive housekeeper from Cindy's childhood, still cranking in her mind. Now that Cindy had accessed this memory/belief, she could use EFT to eliminate it, clearing the way for her positive affirmation to actualize.

Cindy first tapped one round of "Even though I believe I'm a fat pig and always will be, I deeply love and accept myself." I then suggested that she modify the Setup phrase to reenforce her positive affirmation.

She did this by replacing "I deeply love and accept myself" with "I choose to be slim and gorgeous," making her final phrase, "Even though I believe I'm a fat pig and always will be, I choose to be slim and gorgeous."

EFT Affirmation Formula

1. Create your affirmation positively in the present tense, as in "I (fill in your intention, goal, or statement)."
2. Repeat it out loud, listening for your "tail-ender."
3. Insert your tail-ender in your EFT Setup, as in "Even though I (add your tail-ender), I *choose to be* (insert your affirmation)."
4. Repeat the above by tapping a full round of points.

This formula is highly effective because it's authentic. An affirmation always involves making a choice. If you affirm "I am slim . . ." while forty pounds overweight, you are in actuality affirming *the choice* to be slim—beginning right now. This way of doing affirmations strips away what I call the "unreality factor," where a part of you is affirming your new choice while another part of you is contradicting it. It releases the obstacle to your positive intention, while installing it in your body-mind through the power of EFT.

Develop affirmative phrases to add to your EFT Setup. Your affirmations can instill your specific weight-loss or health goal, as in "I choose to be slim forever" or "I choose to enjoy perfect health." They can affirm your ability to adhere to the diet, as in "I crave healthy portions of foods that are good for me and slimming." You can use affirmations to address emotional issues that support weight loss ("I choose to feel worthy" or "I choose to be empowered to make healthy food choices") or to install a positive self-image as in "I choose to be slim, strong, and successful, and weigh 138 pounds."

Using EFT to empower your affirmations is like installing a powerful engine that speeds you toward the actualization of what you want in life, while simultaneously removing all hidden obstacles.

Self-Acceptance

I leave it to your imagination and creativity to seize this wonderful technique and use it to create your hopes and dreams. But if I could elect one belief you should never lack, I'd vote for basic self-acceptance. From all my work with my patients and with myself, this is something I wish for everyone.

My patient Joanne felt deep guilt about her teenage son's accidental death in a motorcycle accident. She was angry at her estranged husband and blamed herself for being so caught up in the drama of her dissolving marriage that she hadn't heard Ryan's cries for help. A recovering alcoholic, Joanne had resumed drinking following Ryan's death. Her downward spiral wasn't helping her, and it isolated Joanne from her fourteen-year-old daughter, Lisa, whose school grades plummeted.

When Joanne did the EFT formula for self-acceptance, it released a flood of tears and almost unbearable grief. But the way out was the way through. Joanne did the formula for three months before she felt the load of self-blame begin to lighten. This enabled her to turn her attention to Lisa, paving the way for mother and daughter to mourn their loss together, an act of healing that freed them both to go forward in life.

No matter where you are in life, no matter what you've contributed to creating, no matter what's happening right now, please remember this. At all times, you are doing the best you can, with the understanding, awareness, and knowledge that you now have. Until you can find a better way to handle the situation, you are doing the best you can. Beating yourself up will never lead you down the right road. Affirming that you are doing your best frees you to move forward to do even better.

Self-Acceptance Formula

1. Create your phrase, using something you feel sadness, pain, guilt, or regret about, as in "Even though (fill in *the situation, experience, behavior, or feelings you feel badly about*) . . ."
2. Add the self-acceptance phrase "I (was/am) doing the best I (could/can)." Repeat the above by tapping a full round of points.

Before you move on from this chapter to the next section of this book, I'd like you to try my self-acceptance formula as my gift to you. Accepting yourself is your birthright. Please don't spend another moment lacking this essential gift.

PART 4

RECIPES

CHAPTER 12

RECIPES

Welcome to a selection of some of my best *No-Grain* recipes. Here are a group of healthy and delicious basics to get you started on the Diet. Some you may already know, while the menu suggestions help you incorporate them according to the principles of this diet. Others may become new favorites that you'll use over and over, and adapt to your own tastes. Others may inspire you with new ideas. Some you may not find to your taste. I urge you to give those that appeal a try, and you may be surprised by the new world of tastes they offer. In particular, if you are starting the Diet in the spring or summer months, I heartily recommend that you give some of the raw juices, salads, soups, and dips a try. Apart from salads, raw cuisine is new to many people, and you'll be surprised at how delicious it can be. It's also a great way to feel satisfied while attaining weight loss!

Breakfast Foods

DR. MERCOLA'S GREEN JUICE DRINK
(with variations)

Your breakfast foundation for Advanced and Core Food Plans

Beginner's Juice Drink:
2 stalks celery
1 cucumber
2 stalks fennel

Put vegetables through a juicer and drink.

Begin with one to two ounces of juice at a time. Gradually, increase until you can drink a twelve-ounce glass of juice. You can prepare several glasses at once, making sure to drink them within the day they are juiced. If you like, on the Advanced Food Plan, you may gradually increase your juice quantities until you are drinking two to three of the twelve-ounce glasses of juice every two hours. To ensure their freshness, store them in the refrigerator in an airtight container (with minimal air space at the top of your container).

Once you are accustomed to juicing, you may add one or more of any of the following, moving from left to right on this chart to incorporate items you enjoy.

Group One	Group Two	Herbs	Flavorings	Protein Powders	Raw Eggs
Mild vegetables: one or more of the following	Strong veggies: begin with two leaves until you are used to them			Rice or whey protein powder**	
1 head red or green leaf lettuce	kale	6 sprigs parsley	1 TBS coconut*	1 to 2 scoops rice or whey protein powder	add one to four eggs (See Resources section for complete instruc- tions.)
½ head romaine lettuce	collard greens	2 TBS cilantro	1 TBS fresh cran- berries		
2 endives	dandelion greens		½ lemon		
½ head escarole	mustard greens (pungent!)		1 inch ginger root		
½ head spinach					
cabbage and Chinese cabbage (start with a few leaves)					

Notes: *Whole fresh grated or unsweetened dry from a health food store
**Recommended rice or whey protein powders are from Metagenics, Nutrabiotics, and other brands recommended on *www.nograindiet.com*

Feel free to experiment and create your own favorite blends. Here are a few examples of tasty combinations:

1. Celery, fennel, cucumber juice with coconut
2. Red leaf, spinach, celery, and raw cranberries
3. Spinach, cucumber, celery, parsley, and ginger root
4. Romaine, dandelion green

SAUSAGE PATTY

Delicious with poached eggs or as a snack
Yield: 8–10 patties

2 pounds lean grass-fed beef or buffalo/bison
1 small onion, finely chopped
1 small green pepper, finely chopped
1 egg, lightly whisked
Celtic sea salt and pepper to taste
Spice option of choice
1 tablespoon olive oil

SPICE MIX OPTIONS:

To flavor your sausage, choose a combination of spices and herbs from these examples; or use your own favorites:

- *Mediterranean*: 1 teaspoon each of thyme, sage, marjoram, and tarragon
- *Italian*: 1 teaspoon each of oregano, thyme, rosemary, and parsley, and ½ teaspoon of chili flakes (optional)
- *Thai*: One-inch lemongrass (finely chopped), 1 tablespoon lime juice plus zest of 1 lime, 1 teaspoon fish sauce,* and ½ teaspoon each of cumin, coriander, ginger, and garlic
- *Jerk*: 3 tablespoons ketchup, 2 tablespoons lime juice, 1 teaspoon soy sauce, 2 teaspoons allspice, and 1 teaspoon each of garlic and cumin

1. Cut the meat into one-inch cubes, then process into ground meat in the food processor (or have a butcher grind the meat for you).
2. In a large bowl, mix the meat, onion, green pepper, egg, salt, pepper, and chosen spices.
3. Form into eight to ten patties. You can cook and freeze them for later use.
4. In a large skillet, cook the patties on medium heat using the olive oil. Cook on each side until nicely browned, ten to fifteen minutes.

*Fish sauce is an Asian sauce made from anchovies that can be found in Asian grocery stores and the ethnic section of many supermarkets.

NO-GRAIN PANCAKES

A special treat for breakfast or brunch
Yield: 4–6 pancakes

5 tablespoons walnuts, ground
½ teaspoon baking powder
2 tablespoons sour cream
1 egg beaten lightly
3 tablespoons water
1 to 2 teaspoons maple extract
1 teaspoon vanilla extract
2 tablespoons oil (choose from butter, ghee, walnut oil, or
   coconut butter)

CINNAMON BUTTER

4 tablespoons softened butter
¾ teaspoon cinnamon

1. In a medium size bowl, mix ground walnuts and baking powder.
2. Add sour cream, egg, water, and extracts. Mix well.
3. Ladle 2 tablespoons of pancake mixture to form each pancake onto preheated and greased (using organic butter, ghee, or coconut butter) frying pan or griddle. Cook on medium heat until golden brown on underside of the pancakes and bubbles form on the top, approximately three to four minutes. Gently turn over and cook for 3 to 4 minutes until golden. Cooled pancakes may be frozen for later use.
4. To make Cinnamon Butter, combine butter and cinnamon and mix until a smooth paste forms. Serve with warm pancakes.

NO-GRAIN MUFFINS

The orange rind makes this recipe yummy
Yield: 6–8 muffins

1 cup flaxseeds, ground
½ cup walnuts, ground
¾ cup protein powder
2 teaspoons baking powder
1 teaspoon baking soda
1 teaspoon cinnamon
½ teaspoon salt
4 teaspoons oil
2 eggs
2 teaspoons vanilla
⅔ cup zucchini, peeled and grated
⅔ cup ricotta cheese
grated zest of one orange
½ cup walnuts, chopped

1. Line muffin tin with paper muffin cups.
2. In a small bowl, mix flaxseeds, walnuts, protein powder, baking powder, baking soda, cinnamon, and salt.
3. In a large bowl, mix oil, eggs, vanilla, grated zucchini, cheese, and orange zest.
4. Fold dry ingredients into liquid ingredients. Fold in chopped walnuts.
5. Pour into muffin tins and bake in a preheated oven at 350 degrees for 20 to 25 minutes.

NO-GRAIN BREAD

Delicious toasted in open-faced sandwiches!
Yield: 7–8 slices

½ cup walnuts, ground
½ cup flaxseeds, ground
1 teaspoon sea salt
5 eggs, separated
¾ cup zucchini, peeled and grated
2 tablespoons walnut oil
¼ teaspoon cream of tartar

1. Line a 10-by-15-inch pan with parchment and grease with olive oil or butter.

2. In a separate bowl, mix walnuts, flaxseeds, and salt.

3. In another bowl, blend egg yolks, zucchini mixture, and walnut oil.

4. Beat egg whites until soft peaks occur. Add cream of tartar and continue beating until stiff but not dry.

5. Fold dry ingredients into egg-yolk mixture. Fold egg whites carefully into egg-yolk mixture and pour into prepared pan and bake in a preheated 350 degree oven for 15 minutes.

6. Cut into 3 ½-by-4-inch squares. Can be frozen for later use.

Appetizers and Snacks

QUICHE

Make this savory treat for breakfast, lunch, and snacks!
Yield: one 8- to 9-inch tart pan, enough for 4–5 portions

QUICHE DOUGH

3-½ cup flaxseeds, ground
¾ cup walnuts, ground
1 teaspoon baking powder
⅔ cup butter, cut into one-inch pieces
2 eggs
1 teaspoon vanilla extract

1. In a medium size bowl or food processor, combine dry ingredients. Add butter and mix until it resembles pea-size crumbs. Don't worry if there are a few larger sized pieces. If mixing dough in bowl, use two forks to work the dough.

2. Add eggs and vanilla extract and mix until the dough is smooth. Form into a ball or flattened circle. If dough is sticky, wrap and refrigerate for ½-hour. Dough can be frozen at this point.

QUICHE BATTER

5 eggs
1 cup whipping cream
1 cup milk
pinch of nutmeg (optional)
½ teaspoon Celtic sea salt
pepper to taste
Optional: spices appropriate to variations
    listed below

1. In a medium-size bowl, whisk eggs lightly. Add all other ingredients including variation flavorings, if wished, and stir to combine.

2. Lightly dust minimal amount of ground flaxseeds onto working surface to prevent dough from sticking to your rolling pin and counter. Roll out dough into a circle of ⅛-inch thickness. Dust off excess flax powder and lift carefully into tart pan. Carefully press dough into pan to fit.

3. If using one of the variations, add vegetables and/or meat directly on top of uncooked quiche dough. Pour quiche batter to fill ¾ up the sides of the quiche.

4. Bake in a preheated 375-degree oven for 30–40 minutes until the surface is slightly golden brown.

Variations:

Leek-Bacon-Garlic: Add roasted garlic, 1 chopped, cooked leek, and cooked turkey bacon on top of rolled-out raw quiche dough. Pour in quiche batter and bake.

Tomato-Thyme: Add to batter 1 teaspoon each of thyme and rosemary. Add ½ cup each raw, sliced zucchini, eggplant, and chopped tomatoes on top of rolled-out raw quiche dough, pour in quiche batter and bake as usual.

Italian Sausage: Add 1 chopped tomato, chopped basil, 1 small finely chopped raw onion, and ½ cup chopped sundried tomatoes (soaked for an hour in warm water) on top of rolled-out raw quiche dough and bake as usual. For Booster, add 1 cooked Italian sausage chopped.

Mushroom-Chicken: Add to batter 1 teaspoon of thyme. Add 1 cup sliced assorted raw mushrooms, 1 cup chopped cooked chicken, and 1 small sautéed onion on top of rolled-out raw quiche dough and bake as directed.

HUMMUS

This Middle-Eastern favorite makes a quick and easy snack!

1⅓ cup dried chickpeas (garbanzo beans)
½ cup tahini (paste from ground sesame seeds)*
3 tablespoons extra-virgin olive oil
5 cloves garlic, finely chopped
¾ teaspoon salt
¼ teaspoon ground cumin
¼ teaspoon cayenne (optional)
½ cup lemon juice
2 tablespoons parsley, chopped (optional)
1 large pinch paprika (optional)

1. Pick over and discard any misshapen peas and stones. Rinse and drain. Cover with water and soak at least four hours, preferably overnight.

2. Drain and discard water. Place in saucepan, cover with 2 inches of water and bring to a boil. Reduce heat and simmer, uncovered, until skins crack and chickpeas are tender, approximately one hour. Drain and reserve liquid.

3. In food processor or blender, combine chickpeas, tahini, olive oil, garlic, salt, cumin, cayenne, and lemon juice to taste. Process until smooth and creamy. If it is too thick, use reserved cooking water to thin it to the desired consistency. Taste and adjust with salt and lemon juice. Sprinkle with parsley and paprika, if desired.

*Tahini can be found in ethnic sections of many grocery stores and in most health food stores.

TANDOORI KABOBS

An Indian spin on kabobs, also great barbecued!

2 cups turkey, uncooked and cut into chunks (you can also use
    chicken, beef, or buffalo/bison)
1 red pepper, cut into chunks
1 small onion, cut into chunks

TANDOORI SPICE MARINADE:

1 teaspoon each chili powder, garlic powder, ground cumin,
    ground ginger, and mild paprika
½ teaspoon each ground cinnamon, saffron (optional), salt,
    and pepper
4 tablespoons grated onion
4–6 tablespoons yogurt
4 tablespoons lemon juice

1. In a large bowl, combine marinade ingredients. Add meat
chunks and marinate at least 2 hours, preferably overnight.
2. If using wooden skewers, to prevent them from burning, soak
them in water for an hour before using. Alternate pieces of meat, onion,
and red pepper on skewers and broil or barbecue on medium heat for
5 to 10 minutes. Turn skewers and broil for another 5 minutes, or until
meat is no longer pink in the center. Beef will take 10 minutes per side
for medium- to well-doneness.
3. Serve with a cool salad and/or dip made of yogurt mixed with
lime juice and mint as this is a hot and spicy dish.

VARIETY ROLL-UP RECIPES

Quick and easy No-Grain snacks

*You can use almost any kind of large, leafy green vegetable to make
great roll-ups, wraps, or nori rolls. You can stuff them with your favorite*

*meat, fish, or poultry along with your favorite vegetables and sauces. This
is a great dish for using up leftovers. Please consult menu plans and
Snack Suggestion list for additional delicious combinations.*

For roll-ups and outer wraps, use as your base:
Leaf, romaine, Boston, or other lettuce
Bok choy, arugala, or collard greens
Cabbage
For nori rolls, use nori seaweed (Sushi Nori by Eden)

Outer wrap	Main Ingredient	Add-ins	Sauce

Romaine, Boston, or other lettuce	Turkey, Chicken	avocado
		baby spinach
		bell peppers
		cucumber
		daikon
		grilled veggies
		scallions
		tomato
		pickles
		sprouts:
		    sunflower,
		    lentil, broccoli
		fresh herbs: basil,
		    cilantro, dill
		cheese*
			Mayonnaise (recipe on p. 214)
			Avocado mayonnaise (recipe on p. 214)
			Walnut Garlic Sauce (recipe on p. 212)
			Pesto (recipe on p. 227)
			mustard
			lemon juice

Lettuces Collard Greens Cabbage	Beef, Buffalo	bell peppers cucumber daikon hot peppers red onion roasted peppers sauerkraut scallions sprouts tomato fresh herbs: basil, cilantro, arugula watercress cheese*	*Mayonnaise* (recipe on p. 214) *Pesto* (recipes on p. 227) hot sauce lime juice horseradish *No-Grain Ketchup* (recipe on p. 215)

(continued)

Outer wrap	Main Ingredient	Add-ins	Sauce

Nori sheets
Collard Greens
Cabbage
	Duck	orange sections
		red onion
		sprouts
		watercress
		radish
		daikon
		scallions
		pickled ginger
		grilled veggies
			Spicy Wasabi
			  Sesame Sauce
			Asian Ginger
			  Sauce
			Roasted Garlic
			  Miso Sauce
			  (recipes on
			  p. 212–213)
			tamari (wheat-
			  free)
			lime juice

Lettuces	Fish and fish salad	tomato
		red onion
		cucumbers
		fresh herbs:
		  dill, tarragon,
		  arugula
		bell peppers
		scallions
		watercress
			Mayonnaise
			  (recipe on p.
			  214)
			Avocado
			  Mayonnaise
			  (recipe on p.
			  214)
			Basil Pesto
			Cilantro
			  Pesto (recipes
			  on p. 227)

*Cheeses for Modified and Core Food Plans: cheddar, Swiss, goat, sheep, Gruyere, Colby, and mozzarella can be used grated or sliced

For Roll-Ups and Wraps

1. Lay the chosen green leaf on a wooden board. You may need to flatten the stem end with the palm of your hand. Cabbage and collard green leaves may be softened for easier rolling by dipping in hot (not boiling) water for 5 minutes and dried thoroughly.

2. Add chosen main ingredient. Top with add-ins and sauce of choice. Add cheese (for Booster or Core Food Plans).

3. Starting at the stem end, roll the leaf tightly, folding in the sides to make the roll-up tight and compact.

Nori Instructions

1. Lay nori sheets on a wooden board.
2. Fill each sheet with choice of main ingredients, add-ins, and sauces.
3. Form nori rolls by tucking in the sides and then rolling the nori sheet away from you.
4. Cut each roll into 3-inch pieces and serve with *Spicy Wasabi Sauce*.

Sauces

For use as dips and condiments with snacks, meats, and vegetables

WALNUT GARLIC SAUCE

¼ cup walnuts, ground
4 garlic cloves, finely chopped
1 tablespoon tamari sauce (wheat-free)
3 tablespoons olive oil

Whisk all ingredients together until smooth.

ROASTED GARLIC MISO SAUCE

8 whole heads garlic
4 tablespoons olive oil
1 teaspoon miso paste
¾ cup hot boiling water

1. Make a miso broth by dissolving 1 teaspoon miso paste in ¾ cup hot water.

2. Remove outer loose skin from garlic heads. Place garlic heads in a baking dish to fit. Pour miso broth around garlic heads and drizzle with olive oil. Bake covered for 1 hour in preheated 400-degree oven. Cool.

3. Squeeze garlic cloves out of garlic head. Mix with ½ cup of the miso broth remaining in the baking dish to make a sauce.

ASIAN GINGER SAUCE

4 green onions, finely chopped
2 tablespoons ginger, finely chopped
1 tablespoon olive oil
1 teaspoon tamari sauce (wheat-free)

Whisk all ingredients together until smooth.

SPICY WASABI SESAME SAUCE

⅓ cup sesame seeds
4 tablespoons tamari sauce (wheat-free)
4 tablespoons water
1 teaspoon lemon juice
1 tablespoon grated ginger
½ teaspoon wasabi powder or to taste

Whisk all ingredients together until smooth.

MAYONNAISE

3 egg yolks
2 tablespoons Dijon mustard
½ teaspoon lemon juice
pinch of sea salt
2 cups olive oil

1. In a medium size bowl, lightly whisk yolks, mustard, lemon juice, and salt together.

2. Slowly drizzle in oil in a small steady stream while continuing to whisk. If the oil is added too quickly, the mayonnaise will not emulsify or thicken. Take your time. This can be done in a blender or food processor but you still must add the oil slowly.

3. Adjust to taste with lemon juice and salt.

Avocado Mayonnaise

Follow main recipe, but add ½ teaspoon lime juice and reduce the lemon juice to ¼ teaspoon. Add 1 pureed avocado before you add the oil.

Dill-Lemon Mayonnaise

Follow main recipe, but increase lemon juice to 1 teaspoon and add grated zest of 1 lemon. Fold in ½ cup of chopped fresh dill after you've blended in the oil.

NO-GRAIN KETCHUP

4 cups tomatoes, chopped
4 onions, chopped
1 red pepper, chopped
1 tablespoon each: allspice, cloves, celery seed, and pepper
1 inch stick of cinnamon
½ teaspoon dry mustard
1 clove garlic
1 bay leaf
1 cup apple cider vinegar

1. Simmer tomatoes, onions, and peppers until soft. Pass through a strainer to catch skins. If you don't have a good strainer, peel the tomatoes first. Measure the amount of tomato mixture.

2. Add spices and bring to boil, stirring often. Continue cooking until mixture is reduced to one-half of the amount you measured. Add vinegar and simmer 10 minutes. Add salt and cayenne to taste.

Soup

BASIC CREAM SOUP
WITH VARIATIONS

This soup is the foundation for many variations,
using your favorite vegetables
Yield: 5 portions

2 tablespoons olive oil
4 cloves garlic, finely chopped
1 large onion, chopped
1 stalk celery, chopped
3 cups chopped vegetables of choice:
   broccoli florets,
   asparagus (tough ends removed)
   mushrooms
   spinach (tough stems removed)
   zucchini
   tomato (skin and seeds removed*)
4 cups chicken broth
2 cups water
1 teaspoon thyme
1 teaspoon parsley
Celtic sea salt and pepper to taste
¼ cup ground flaxseeds
1 cup heavy cream (or if non-dairy, ¾ cup unsweetened
   coconut milk**)
1 tablespoon chives, chopped

1. In a soup pot, sauté garlic, onion, and celery in olive oil on low heat for about five minutes. Add vegetable of choice and sauté for five minutes.

2. Add broth, water, herbs, salt, and pepper to pot and simmer covered for 20–30 minutes.

3. Cool soup before adding ground flaxseeds and pureeing in a blender in batches.

4. Add heavy cream gradually, stirring with wire whisk to ensure smoothness.

5. Heat gently on low before serving. Garnish with chives.

Variations

Creamy Cheese and Vegetable Soup: After whisking in cream, warm the soup and add ½ cup grated organic cheddar or Gruyere cheese.

Asparagus Leek Soup: Use asparagus as vegetable of choice and replace onion with two chopped leeks.

Creamy Curry Soup: Use spinach as vegetable of choice and omit garlic. Omit thyme and parsley, replacing them with 1 teaspoon turmeric, ½ teaspoon each ginger and coriander, and ¼ teaspoon cayenne (optional). For Sustain version, garnish with 1 tablespoon of sweet peas.

Carrot Zucchini Soup (Sustain Phase only): For vegetables, use 2 cups of zucchini and 1 cup of diced carrots. Omit garlic and onion; replace with 2 diced scallions. Omit parsley, thyme, and chives, and season with 1 teaspoon pumpkin pie spice mix.

*To easily remove tomato skins, cut an "X" in the bottom of tomatoes and briefly dip into boiling water. Cool and peel.

**Please check the label to ensure that no sweetener or corn syrup is contained in the product.

Raw Foods and Salads

ENERGY SOUP

A tangy way to eat your vegetables!
Yield: 4 portions

1 cucumber, peeled and chopped
½ bunch spinach, rinsed, stems removed, and torn into pieces
5 tablespoons lemon or lime juice
2 tablespoons minced ginger root
1 tablespoon minced garlic
4 sprigs parsley
½ cup sprouts: sunflower, broccoli, or, for the Booster Food
    Plan, lentil or mung bean
Celtic sea salt to taste
⅛ teaspoon cayenne pepper
1½ cups water
1 avocado, peeled with pit removed
½ cup cilantro, chopped
2 scallions, chopped

1. In a food processor, puree the cucumber, spinach, lemon juice, ginger, garlic, parsley, sprouts, salt, and cayenne. Add avocado and blend allowing some small pieces to remain. If soup is too thick, you can add more cucumber or water.

2. Stir in cilantro and scallions and refrigerate until ready to serve.

Variations

Broccoli Sprout Energy Soup: Replace sunflower sprouts with broccoli sprouts. Reduce water to 1 cup. Omit ginger. Add 2 tablespoons organic coconut oil for creaminess, and flavor with chopped, fresh dill instead of cilantro.

Mint Watercress Energy Soup: Omit spinach, garlic, and sprouts. Use ½ bunch watercress, ½ cup chopped mint, and proceed as instructed. Garnish with a cherry tomato.

Midsummer Gazpacho Energy Soup: Soak three organic sun-dried tomatoes for 1 hour in ½ cup water. Drain and save water. Reserve ½ cup of the chopped cuke for serving. Puree remaining cucumber pieces and process as instructed, omitting spinach, ginger, avocado, and decreasing water to ½ cup. Add 1 cup chopped cherry tomatoes, drained sun-dried tomatoes, tomato water, and ¼ cup chopped basil. Blend. Add 1 to 2 tablespoons of chopped cuke to each bowl, add soup, and garnish with yellow pepper slices.

Sunshine Energy Soup (for Sustain phase only): Omit garlic, scallions, and pepper. First puree ⅔ cup of pineapple with cucumber until smooth. Use sunflower sprouts and proceed as instructed, saving the avocado and cilantro until last, and only mixing slightly. Top with toasted unsweetened coconut.

Harvest Energy Soup (for Sustain phase only): Soak 3 tablespoons of flaxseeds in ½ cup water overnight. Next day, puree ⅔ cup of chopped peeled apples with cucumber until smooth. Omit spinach, garlic, scallions, and pepper. Add flaxseeds and water mixture. Use sunflower sprouts and proceed as instructed, saving the avocado until last.

MULTICOLORED COLESLAW

A favorite salad, four ways!

½ **head red cabbage, shredded**
½ **head green cabbage, shredded**
½ **red onion, chopped**
1 **zucchini, thinly sliced**
juice of a lemon
Celtic sea salt to taste
1 **tablespoon natural mustard**
¾ **cup *Mayonnaise* (recipe on page 214) or ½ cup olive oil**

1. Shred vegetables by hand or use a food processor.

2. Combine lemon juice, salt, mustard, and mayonnaise or olive oil and pour over vegetables.

3. Refrigerate to develop flavors for about two hours.

Variations

Dilly Slaw: Replace red onion with ⅓ cup chopped scallions. Add ¼ cup chopped dill, 1 finely sliced radish and 1 tablespoon caraway seeds.

Asian Slaw: Omit mustard, salt, and lemon juice. Shred a 2-inch piece of daikon and add to mix. Add 3 tablespoons rice vinegar and 1 tablespoon soy sauce. Sprinkle with sesame seeds.

Mexican Slaw: Omit zucchini and mustard, and replace with 1 thinly sliced red pepper, 1 chopped jalapeño pepper*, (optional) and ¼ cup chopped black olives. Add ¼ cup of sour cream to mayonnaise and fold in ¼ cup of chopped cilantro, and 2 tablespoons lime juice. Season with a sprinkle of red pepper flakes.

*Note: Handle jalapeño with gloves, and rinse carefully after handling to avoid burning your skin or eyes.

Main Dishes

ASIAN CHICKEN SALAD

A cool summer salad
Yield: 4–5 servings

2 pounds chicken, cut into chunks (you can use turkey,
  salmon, tilapia, or duck)
2 tablespoons olive or walnut oil
1 cucumber, sliced
½ red onion, sliced
½ cup fresh mint, lightly chopped

½ cup bean sprouts
sprouts for garnish
Salad Greens for 4–5 servings

DRESSING:

½ cup lime juice
4 tablespoons fish sauce*
¼ cup olive or walnut oil
1 stalk lemongrass, finely chopped**
2-inch piece of ginger, finely chopped
1 clove garlic, crushed
2 tablespoons cilantro, chopped
½ teaspoon chili flakes
4 tablespoons of chopped almonds (Booster Food Plan only)

1. Baste chicken with oil. Place on grill or in preheated 400-degree oven. Grill or broil until tender and cooked through, about 10 minutes. Cool.

2. Assemble dressing ingredients.

3. Toss salad greens in a small amount of the dressing and arrange on plates.

4. Toss remaining ingredients in the dressing and arrange on top of lettuce.

5. Garnish with sprouts. For Booster Food Plan, sprinkle 4 table-spoons of chopped almonds over salad.

*Fish sauce is an Asian sauce made from anchovies that can be found in Asian grocery stores and in the ethnic section of many supermarkets.

**Lemongrass can be found in Asian grocery stores and in the ethnic section of many supermarkets.

PEPPER STEAK

A great way to enjoy grass-fed beef!
Yield: 3–4 portions

2 tablespoons salt
1 pound grass-fed beef or buffalo/bison strip loin
¼ cup peppercorns, crushed roughly
¼ cup butter
1 teaspoon tamari sauce (wheat-free)
2 tablespoons beef stock
2 tablespoons lemon juice

1. Place peppercorns on a plate and press steak into peppercorns to cover both sides thickly. Work peppercorns into meat with your hands.

2. Sprinkle a skillet with the salt and over medium heat, cook until salt begins to brown. Add steak to the pan and brown over high heat. Reduce to medium heat and cook until it reaches desired degree of doneness, approximately 3–4 minutes per side for medium-rare. Discard drippings.

3. In a separate saucepan, combine butter, tamari, beef stock, and lemon juice.

4. Serve the steak with the sauce on the side.

HEARTY STEW

This scrumptious classic can be prepared with your favorite meat!
Yield: 6–8 dinner-sized portions

6 slices turkey bacon, sliced and cut vertically in small strips
2 cloves garlic, sliced
12 small onions, whole, peeled
1 cup celery, chopped
1 cup red pepper, chopped
2 cups button mushrooms, whole

1 ounce dried mushrooms, preferably porcini, or any dried
   mushroom, rinsed of dirt (optional)
2 pounds lean, boneless stewing beef, buffalo, or veal, cut into
   chunks
2 tablespoons paprika
2 tablespoons flaxseeds, ground
2 cups beef broth
1 bay leaf
½ teaspoon pepper
sea salt to taste
1 cup parsley, chopped

1. Soak the mushrooms in hot beef broth or water for 1 hour.
Drain (reserving the liquid) and chop the mushrooms.

2. Sauté bacon slices in a large pot over medium-low heat. Drain
off excess fat. Add garlic, onions, celery, red pepper, and button mushrooms and continue to sauté for 10 minutes. Set vegetables aside.

3. Roll meat in paprika and ground flaxseeds and add to pot. Sauté
until brown and cooked through.

4. Return vegetables to pot. Add stock, chopped, rehydrated mushrooms and their liquid, bay leaf, salt, pepper, and parsley. Simmer for 1
hour. Add more stock if needed.

No-Grain Pastas

Enjoy your favorite pasta dishes grain-free

ZUCCHINI "LASAGNA"

Yield: 6 dinner-size portions

6–7 zucchini squash
2 cups ricotta cheese
pinch of nutmeg
1 pound raw spinach, steamed for 1 minute or 1 cup fresh
  basil, chopped
1 pound grated organic mozzarella cheese
Tomato Meat Sauce **(recipe follows)**

1. Mix the ricotta cheese, nutmeg, and steamed spinach or basil. Set aside.

2. Spread about ¼ cup of meat sauce over bottom of a 9-by-13-inch baking pan.

3. Cover with a single layer of ⅓ of the zucchini "pasta." (See page 225.)

4. Scatter ⅓ of the ricotta cheese mixture over the zucchini "pasta."

5. Add ¼ of the remaining tomato meat sauce, followed by ⅓ the mozzarella cheese. This makes 1 full layer.

6. Continue for 2 more layers, using remaining zucchini, ricotta, meat sauce, and mozzarella in that order. Make sure to finish with mozzarella.

7. Bake at 375 degrees for 20–25 minutes. Let stand 10 minutes before cutting.

VARIATION: CONFETTI PASTA

Yield: 4–5 dinner-sized portions

3 tablespoons olive oil
2 garlic cloves, finely chopped

¼ teaspoon dried oregano
1 red pepper, thinly sliced
1 yellow or orange pepper, thinly sliced
6 zucchini squash
Celtic sea salt and pepper
Tomato Meat Sauce (recipe follows)

1. In a skillet, heat oil over medium heat. Sauté garlic in 2 tablespoons olive oil for 30 seconds. Add peppers and oregano and sauté until cooked, but not limp, approximately 5 minutes. Set aside.

2. Prepare sauce. (See recipes for *Tomato Meat Sauce* and *Walnut Basil Pesto* on page 227.)

3. While the sauce cooks, prepare zucchini "pasta." Using a vegetable peeler or a very sharp knife, shave zucchini lengthwise into long, thin pasta-like strips. Spread in a single layer on an oiled cookie sheet, brush lightly with olive oil, and season lightly with sea salt and pepper. Bake for 5 minutes in a 425-degree oven.

5. Toss zucchini and peppers with *Walnut Pesto* or *Tomato Meat Sauce*; for Booster or Core Food Plan, serve with organic cheddar or parmesan cheese (optional).

Sustain Diet Variation: SPAGHETTI SQUASH SPAGHETTI

Yield: 2 dinner-sized portions

1 spaghetti squash
2 cups *Tomato Meat Sauce* (recipe follows)

1. To cook spaghetti squash, cut squash in half lengthwise. Remove seeds and place cut side down in a baking dish. Pour 1 cup water around squash halves. Bake squash for one hour at 350 degrees. Cool slightly.

2. During baking, prepare sauce.

3. Pull the squash from its shell with a fork. It will come out in "spaghetti" type strands. Top with sauce.

Pasta Sauces

TOMATO MEAT SAUCE

Yield: approximately 2 quarts

2 tablespoons olive oil
4 cloves garlic, finely chopped
1 cup onion, chopped
½ cup green pepper, chopped
1½ pounds ground grass-fed beef, lamb, or buffalo meat
1 cup mushrooms, sliced
1 13-ounce can tomatoes, chopped
1 6-ounce can tomato paste
2 teaspoons dried basil
1 teaspoon dried oregano
1 teaspoon dried thyme
1 bay leaf
½ teaspoon red chili flakes
1 teaspoon red wine vinegar
Celtic sea salt to taste

1. Heat oil in a large heavy pot over medium low heat. Sauté garlic in 2 tablespoons olive oil for 30 seconds. Add onion and green pepper and cook until onion is translucent and peppers are partially cooked.
2. Add ground meat of choice and cook until browned. Drain pan drippings.
3. Stir in mushrooms, spices, tomatoes, and tomato paste.
4. Simmer for 40 minutes, stirring occasionally. If it becomes too thick for your taste, add ½ cup of water. Remove bay leaf.
5. Add vinegar and salt. Adjust seasoning according to taste.

Pestos

Delicious with "pasta," roll-ups, and vegetables!
Yield 1 cup

WALNUT BASIL

2 cups basil leaves, rinsed
2 cloves garlic, finely chopped
½ cup walnuts
½ cup extra-virgin olive oil
Celtic sea salt and pepper to taste

1. In a food processor or blender, add basil, garlic, and walnuts. Gradually pour olive oil in a steady, thin stream through the chute of the food processor until the pesto emulsifies. Add salt and pepper.

CILANTRO PESTO

Follow the basic recipe, substituting cilantro for basil

ARUGULA PESTO

Follow the basic recipe, substituting arugula for basil
and increasing garlic to 3 cloves

SUNDRIED TOMATO PESTO

6 organic sundried tomatoes
½ cup warm water
3 cloves garlic, finely chopped
½ cup spinach leaves
½ cup walnuts
½ cup extra-virgin olive oil
Celtic sea salt and pepper to taste

1. Soak sun-dried tomatoes for 1 hour in ½ cup water. Drain and discard water.

2. In a food processor or blender, add tomatoes, garlic, spinach, and walnuts. Gradually pour olive oil in a steady, thin stream through the chute of the food processor until the pesto emulsifies. Add salt and pepper.

SOUTHWESTERN CHILI

This classic chili is great with your favorite meat
Yield: 6–8 dinner-size portions

2 tablespoons olive oil
1–2 cloves, garlic, finely chopped
2 large onions, chopped
1 green pepper, chopped
1 cup mushrooms, sliced
1½ pounds ground grass-fed beef, buffalo, ostrich, or tempeh*
1 bay leaf
2 tablespoons chili powder
2 tablespoons ground cumin
1 tablespoon dried oregano
¼ teaspoon ground allspice
pinch of red chili flakes
2 16-ounce cans tomatoes, with liquid

2 cans kidney beans
Sea salt to taste
2 tablespoons fresh parsley, chopped
2 tablespoons fresh cilantro, chopped
3 scallions, thinly slivered on the diagonal

1. Heat the oil in a large heavy pot over medium-low heat. Add garlic, onions, green peppers, and mushrooms. Cook, stirring occasionally, until vegetables have wilted, about 10 minutes.

2. Add ground meat and cook until browned. Add spices and toss to cover meat well.

3. Add tomatoes and their liquid and simmer 30 minutes. Add beans and simmer 30 minutes more. Add salt. Adjust seasoning according to taste.

4. Serve garnished with scallions, parsley, and cilantro.

*If using tempeh, you can remove the bitterness by mixing two tablespoons olive oil and two tablespoons soy sauce into 1 cup of vegetable broth along with the finely chopped garlic cloves. Pour this mixture over the tempeh and braise in a 350-degree oven for 20–30 minutes or until browned. Discard liquid. Crumble tempeh with fork to simulate ground meat.

BOMBAY CURRY

Enjoy these subtle Indian flavors with your choice of meat
Yield: 6–8 dinner-sized portions

2 tablespoons butter, ghee, or olive oil
2 onions, chopped
2 cloves garlic, finely chopped
2 tablespoons ginger root, grated
2 tablespoons curry powder
1 tablespoon ground cumin
1 teaspoon ground coriander
2 pounds grass-fed beef or buffalo meat, cut into chunks
1 medium cauliflower, cut into florets
2 cups vegetable broth
1 16-ounce can tomatoes, chopped
2 cups plain yogurt
1 can chickpeas or 1 cup dry (see *Hummus* recipe on p. 208
   for cooking directions)
Celtic sea salt to taste

1. Heat the oil in a large heavy pot over medium-low heat. Add garlic and onion and cook until wilted, for 8–10 minutes, stirring occasionally. Add spices and cook for 2–3 minutes to coat onions and roast spices well.

2. Add meat and cook until browned. Add cauliflower, vegetable broth, and tomatoes with their juices. Simmer 20 minutes. Add chickpeas and simmer 10 more minutes. Add yogurt just before serving. Don't worry when the yogurt separates and becomes grainy. It still tastes delicious. Add salt and adjust seasoning according to taste.

THAI CHICKEN CURRY

Use the same ingredients in Bombay Curry, but omit chickpeas and replace meat with chicken. For spices, omit curry and add 1–2 green or red chilies, 1 stalk lemongrass*, all finely chopped. Wear gloves in handling chilies and *avoid contact with eyes. Substitute 2 cans of coconut milk for tomatoes. Add 2 tablespoons fish sauce**, ½ cup each of chopped fresh cilantro and bean sprouts. Garnish with chopped almonds.*

*Lemongrass can be found in Asian grocery stores and the ethnic section of many supermarkets.

**Fish sauce is an Asian sauce made from anchovies that can be found in Asian grocery stores and the ethnic section of many supermarkets.

CREAMY FISH CAKES*

A treat from the sea, good for a meal or a snack!
Yield: 8 dinner-sized cakes

¼ cup scallion, finely chopped
3 cloves garlic, finely chopped
1 tablespoon ginger, finely chopped
1 green chili, finely chopped
1 teaspoon grated lemon zest
1¼ pound fish (flounder, salmon, tilapia, or other seafood from Booster Food Plan)
⅔ cup *Mayonnaise* (see recipe on p. 214)
1 cup flaxseed, ground
2 tablespoons oil

1. Combine all ingredients except flaxseed and form into patties. Gently press fish cakes into ground flaxseed to cover all sides.
2. Heat oil in a skillet on medium-high heat. Sauté cakes gently 3–4 minutes per side until golden brown and cooked through. Serve with yogurt mixed with ¼ cup of cilantro, mint, and lime juice.

*I generally avoid consuming fish because most are now showing high mercury toxicity. Please make sure your fish has been lab tested and shown to be free of detectable levels of mercury and other toxins.

Vegetables

STIR-FRIED VEGETABLES

A new twist on a healthy standard

2 tablespoons olive oil
2 cloves garlic, finely chopped
1 inch piece ginger, finely chopped
1 scallion, thinly sliced on the diagonal
1 stalk celery, thinly sliced
½ head broccoli, cut into florets
½ head cauliflower, cut into florets
½ head bok choy, thinly sliced on the diagonal
½ red pepper, thinly sliced
½ cup snow peas
4 mushrooms, sliced
2 tablespoons tamari sauce (wheat-free)
½ teaspoon chili flakes
4 tablespoons chicken stock or water
1 tablespoon kuzu*, dissolved in 4 tablespoons cold water

1. In a wok or large skillet, sauté scallions, garlic, and ginger on low heat for 1 minute.

2. Add celery, broccoli, cauliflower, bok choy, and red pepper. Sauté on medium-high heat, stirring constantly, until vegetables are halfway cooked.

3. Add snow peas and mushrooms and continue to cook for 2–3 more minutes.

4. Add tamari, chili flakes, chicken stock, and kuzu dissolved in water. Bring to a boil and reduce sauce until vegetables are glazed and shiny, 3–4 minutes.

Other vegetable choices include asparagus, zucchini, eggplant, endive, cabbage, a variety of different mushrooms, string beans, torn collard greens, or other greens. Sprouts are a great addition, stirred in at end to avoid overcooking.

Note: Kuzu is an Asian vegetable thickener available at health food stores and Asian markets.

CAULIFLOWER MASHERS WITH GRAVY

Missing mashed potatoes? Try these!

1 head cauliflower, chopped into florets
¼ cup heavy cream or milk
Sea salt and pepper to taste
pinch of nutmeg

1. Steam cauliflower until tender, about 15 minutes.
2. Puree in a food processor with the cream or milk, salt, pepper and nutmeg, adding more cream if necessary.

GRAVY

2 tablespoons olive oil
1 clove garlic, finely chopped
1 teaspoon each thyme and rosemary
½ teaspoon sage
¼ teaspoon paprika
Celtic sea salt and pepper, to taste
½ pound mushrooms, sliced
¾ cup vegetable stock or water
1 tablespoon tamari sauce (wheat-free)
2 tablespoons kuzu*, dissolved in ¼ cup cold water

1. In a skillet, sauté garlic, herbs, salt, pepper, and mushrooms in olive oil until wilted.
2. Add the stock, tamari, and kuzu dissolved in water and bring to boil, stirring constantly.
5. Reduce heat, stirring constantly, until gravy has thickened.
6. Serve gravy over cauliflower "mashers."

Note: Kuzu is an Asian vegetable thickener available at health food stores and Asian markets.

Sustain Recipes

Once you have made it to Sustain, you can continue to build upon the repertory of foods you've learned to enjoy in Start-Up and Stabilize, while slowly transitioning through grain reintroduction. The key to the Sustain phase is maintaining your weight loss and health, while gradually reintroducing modest amounts of healthy grains, starchy vegetables, and selected fruits and desserts. The recipes in this section are your road map in learning how to navigate at safe levels. Consult the menu plans in Chapter Eight to assure that you eat these foods only occasionally, and monitor your portions wisely.

OVEN BAKED YAM OR KOHLRABI CHIPS

Crispy chips for Sustain Diet only

1 raw yam or kohlrabi per person (approximately)
1 onion, thinly sliced
olive oil
sea salt

1. Slice raw yam or kohlrabi into thin "chips" ⅛- to ¼-inch thick.
2. Arrange slices in a single layer or slightly overlapping in a large baking pan and scatter onion slices on top. Brush with olive oil and sprinkle with sea salt.
3. Bake at 375 degrees for 30–45 minutes or until crispy.

Grains
Sustain Only

Follow the basic instructions on how to prepare whole grains, which can be used to make pilafs, cereals, and other dishes. Seek out recipes from other sources. When in doubt, a dash of olive oil, Celtic salt, and parsley tastes good on any grain. Use this chart to guide you in amounts and cooking times.

Grain 1 cup dry	Water (cups)	Time (in minutes)
Brown rice Short grain Long grain	 2 ½	 40 35
Millet	2	25
Amaranth	3	30
Teff	4	20
Oats	2	20
Quinoa	2	15

You will need slightly more water if you cook three or more cups of grain. Also consider whether you prefer your grain dish more wet or more dry. If you prefer a moister grain, add ½ cup more water.

To prepare, bring grain, salt, and water to a boil. Cover and reduce heat to simmer for the time given. Garnish with suggestions listed below.

Grains are delicious when topped with any of these garnishes: chopped parsley or herbs of choice, lemon zest, organic butter, organic coconut butter, toasted sesame seeds, toasted unsweetened coconut, chopped scallions, chopped walnuts, chopped turkey bacon, wheat-free tamari soy sauce, hot sauce, or shredded organic cheese.

VEGETABLE PILAF

You can use any grain in this delicious pilaf
Yield: 6–8 portions

2 tablespoons butter
2 medium onions, chopped
2 tablespoons garlic, finely chopped
2 tablespoons ginger, finely chopped
1 cinnamon stick
2 whole cloves
1½ cups basmati rice
½ cup of fresh peas
3 cups vegetable stock or water

1. Heat the butter in a saucepan. Add the onions, garlic, ginger, cinnamon, cloves. Cook until vegetables wilt slightly, approximately 10 minutes.

2. Add the rice and cook, stirring, for about 1 minute.

3. Add the peas and broth and bring to boil. Reduce the heat to low and simmer covered until the rice is cooked and the liquid has been absorbed, about 10–15 minutes. Fluff with a fork and serve.

Variations

Brown Rice Pilaf: 45 minutes

Millet Pilaf: 25 minutes

Healthy Desserts
Booster and Core Food Plans Only

Now that you've rebalanced your insulin response and reeducated your tastebuds, if you're on the Booster or Core Food Plans, you are ready to enjoy these dessert recipes. Desserts don't have to be harmful if they are prepared with healthy ingredients and eaten rarely *and* in small portions. Nor should you eat desserts every day of the week. Consider them a rare treat, unless you are exercising vigorously every day!

Since the amount of sugar in American desserts has progressively risen over time, my *No-Grain* desserts are less sweet than what you are used to. Yet they are truly delicious and are based on the types of desserts that Europeans have relished for centuries.

Please make sure that when preparing them you do not exceed the recommended amount of sweetener, or use any sweetener not allowed on this diet. Try recipes first by using less sweet fruits such as plums, strawberries, and Granny Smith apples before going on to try sweeter fruits, like peaches or apricots. Remember to eat very small portions and to keep track of the impact these sweeter foods have on you. Please don't eat them at all if they trigger cravings, energy dives, or weight gain. But if you find you can consume small portions safely—enjoy!

The smoothies and salads are refreshing treats in summer while the baked fruits and crumbles are tasty in cooler weather. You can enjoy my *No-Grain Fruit Pie* with summer fruits and a dab of whipped cream. The *Old Europe Walnut Torte* is a typical Viennese dessert, very rich, with flavors that enhance with time.

Fresh Raw Fruit Desserts

FRUIT SMOOTHIES

Creamy and invigorating!

BASIC SMOOTHIE RECIPE

1 cup plain yogurt, heavy cream, or unsweetened coconut milk
**2 cups fresh or frozen fruit, cut into bite-sized pieces, with
peels, pits, and seeds removed**

Combine all ingredients into a blender and blend until smooth.

Variations

1. Fruit variations to use in basic recipe:

1½ cups blueberries or strawberries and 1 banana
2 nectarines or peaches, 1 banana, and 1 kiwi
1 cup grapes, 2 kiwi, 1 nectarine, and 2 apricots
½ cantaloupe, ½ cup fresh coconut, and 1 orange
1 cup raspberries, 2 kiwi, and 2 apples
1 cup apricots, ½ cup raspberries, and 2 kiwi

2. For a thicker consistency, add 6–8 ice cubes before blending, or prefreeze the fruit in bite-sized pieces.
3. Place the blended smoothie in dessert cups and freeze 2 hours before eating.
4. For a higher protein snack, add 1 tablespoon protein powder (whey or rice) before blending.
5. Add ¼ teaspoon organic alcohol-free extract such as vanilla, orange, or almond.
6. Add 2 tablespoons organic unsweetened nut butter for extra protein, flavor, and thickness.

Follow the basic recipe to prepare these delicious smoothies:

COCONUT-APRICOT SMOOTHIE

1 cup unsweetened coconut milk
2 cups fresh apricots, frozen
2 kiwi, frozen

MELBA SMOOTHIE

1 cup plain yogurt
1 cup peaches, frozen
1 cup raspberries, frozen
½ teaspoon grated ginger root

MANGO MINT

1 cup plain yogurt
1 cup mangoes, frozen
1 peach, frozen
1 tablespoon fresh, chopped mint

KIWI-STRAWBERRY

1 cup unsweetened coconut milk
2 kiwi, frozen
1½ cups frozen strawberries
2 tablespoons unsweetened grated coconut
¼ teaspoon organic almond extract

Baked Fruit Desserts

BAKED APPLES

An old favorite!

6 firm Granny Smith apples
2 tablespoons butter, softened
2 tablespoons maple syrup or 1 teaspoon stevia powder*
2 tablespoons cinnamon
6 tablespoons walnuts, chopped
2 tablespoons oats (optional)
½ cup water
1 cup whipped cream or plain yogurt (optional)

*Stevia powder is a natural sweetener available at health food stores.

1. Using a melon-baller or small spoon and starting from the bottom of the apple, core ¾ of the way up to the stem. Place apples in baking dish.

2. In a bowl, combine butter, maple syrup or stevia powder, cinnamon, walnuts, and oats, if desired.

3. Put a few teaspoons of the mixture in holes in cored apples.

4. Pour water around apples.

5. Bake at 350 degrees, covered, for 40 to 50 minutes or until tender.

6. Serve hot or cold, plain, with fresh whipped cream or plain yogurt.

Variations

1. Add 1 tablespoon grated orange or lemon zest to mixture before filling cored apples.

2. Add 2 tablespoons sesame tahini paste to mixture before filling cored apples.

3. Substitute pears, peaches, or plums for the apples.

To prepare pears: core from the bottom only using a melon-baller or small spoon. Fill cavity with filling. Reduce cook time to 20 minutes.

To prepare peaches or plums: cut them in half and take out the pit. Fill cavity with filling. Reduce cook time to 20 minutes.

NO-GRAIN FRUIT TART

Try it with summer fruit, or at any time!

FILLING

4 cups sliced fruit (such as apples, pears, peaches, plums, or
    berries)
2 tablespoons lemon juice
1 teaspoon organic alcohol-free vanilla extract
1 tablespoon cinnamon or to taste
2 tablespoons maple syrup or 2 teaspoons stevia powder*

CRUST

1¼ cup walnuts, ground
2 tablespoons stevia powder*
1¼ cup flaxseed, ground
⅛ teaspoon salt
1 tablespoon baking powder
1 egg, lightly beaten
⅓ cup butter, softened
¼ cup flaxseed, ground

1. Preheat oven to 350 degrees.
2. Combine dry ingredients and mix well. Add egg and butter and mix until well incorporated. Cool in refrigerator for 30 minutes.
3. In a bowl, mix sliced fruit, lemon juice, vanilla, and maple syrup or stevia powder. Allow to rest to infuse flavors for 15 to 30 minutes.
4. Sprinkle flaxseed on your working surface. Use as little as possible, just enough to ensure dough does not stick. Roll out dough to ⅛-inch thickness and fit into 9-inch tart or pie pan. Add fruit and bake for 40 to 50 minutes or until apples are tender.
5. Serve warm or cold, plain, with whipped cream, or plain yogurt.

Variations

1. Fruit suggestions: Use Granny Smith type of apple. If you use pears, peaches, plums, or berries, reduce sweetener to 1 tablespoon of maple syrup or stevia powder.
2. Substitute vanilla with 1 teaspoon grated fresh ginger root (good with pears).
3. Sprinkle tart with ⅔ cup sesame seeds or chopped walnuts after the first 20 minutes of baking. Bake for an additional 10 minutes.

*Stevia powder is a natural sweetener available at health food stores.

NO-GRAIN FRUIT CRUMBLE

Hearty and healthy!

4 cups sliced fruit (apples, pears, peaches, plums, or berries)
2 tablespoons lemon juice
1 teaspoon organic, alcohol-free vanilla extract
1 tablespoon cinnamon
2 tablespoons maple syrup or 1 teaspoon stevia powder*

CRUMBLE TOPPING

⅓ cup walnuts, chopped
⅓ cup oats
¼ cup flaxseed, ground
8 tablespoons butter, softened
½ teaspoon organic, alcohol-free vanilla extract
2 tablespoons maple syrup or 2 tablespoons stevia powder*

1. In a bowl, mix sliced fruit, lemon juice, vanilla, cinnamon, and maple syrup or stevia powder. Pour into a 2-inch deep baking dish.
2. Mix the topping ingredients with a fork until crumbly.
3. Spread the topping over the fruit mixture. Bake at 350 degrees for 40 to 45 minutes.

*Stevia powder is a natural sweetener available at health food stores.

MERINGUE SWIRL COOKIES

Light and meltingly tasty!

BASIC RECIPE

3 egg whites
¼ teaspoon cream of tartar

½ **teaspoon organic, alcohol-free vanilla extract (or almond, coffee, or lemon extract)**
2 teaspoon rice syrup*

1. Preheat oven to 300 degrees.
1. Place the egg whites, cream of tartar, and extract in a medium-size bowl.
2. Beat the egg-white mixture with a wire whisk or electric beaters until the egg whites stand up in firm peaks.
3. Slowly add the rice syrup or stevia powder, continuing to beat until the sweetener is well incorporated into the egg whites.
4. Drop cone-shaped tablespoons of egg-white mixture onto a parchment-lined baking sheet.
5. Bake for 12–15 minutes or until firm.

Variations

1. *Coconut*: Fold in ½ cup unsweetened coconut and substitute vanilla extract with ½ teaspoon of alcohol-free coconut extract.
2. *Walnut*: Fold in ½ cup finely chopped walnuts and substitute vanilla for ½ teaspoon of walnut oil.
3. *Orange*: Add 1 tablespoon orange rind and substitute vanilla extract with ½ teaspoon of alcohol-free orange extract.
4. *Sesame*: Fold in 1 tablespoon tahini** and sprinkle sesame seeds on top of each meringue before baking.
5. *Mocha*: Fold in 1 tablespoon carob powder*** and replace vanilla extract with ½ teaspoon coffee extract.

*Rice syrup is available at health food stores.
**Tahini can be found at health food and Middle-Eastern stores.
***Carob powder is available at health food stores.

OLD EUROPE WALNUT TORTE

A Viennese classic with a new twist!

12 eggs, separated
¾ cup maple syrup
1 lemon, zest and juice
½ cup flaxseeds, ground
6 cups walnuts, ground but not too fine

1. Boil maple syrup until you have 5 tablespoons. Keep warm.

2. Whip egg yolks until thick and pale yellow. While continuing to whip, pour in maple syrup while still warm and runny. If maple syrup hardens, add 1 tablespoon of water. Return to stove and heat until you have a thick syrup.

3. Add lemon rind, juice, and ground flaxseeds to yolk and maple syrup mixture.

4. In separate bowl, beat egg whites until firm but not dry.

5. Gently fold egg whites and nuts into yolk mixture, taking care not to over fold.

6. Pour batter into well-buttered 9-inch spring-form pan and bake in preheated 350-degree oven for 25 to 30 minutes until center springs back when lightly touched. Cool.

7. Carefully slice torte into two layers. You can then fill the layers with any of the three variations of fillings below.

Variations: Grated orange rind and juice may be substituted for grated lemon.

Note: Always store your torte in its spring-form pan in the refrigerator and wrap tightly to preserve its freshness.

Torte Fillings

This torte is delicious with both layers sandwiched together with a thin layer of *Fruit Filling*, *Chantilly Cream*, or *Buttercream* (recipes below). You can also combine a fruit filling with one of the cream fillings.

Note: Chantilly Cream will only last one day in the refrigerator before it starts to "weep," so if you're serving the torte the next day, serve the cream on the side.

FRUIT FILLING

**2 cups any fruit, pureed, and seeds removed (berries work
    very well)**
Sweetener to taste, either maple syrup or stevia
½ cup juice or water
4 tablespoons agar-agar flakes*

1. Mix the juice or water with the agar-agar flakes. Bring to a boil. Reduce heat to low and continue to cook until the agar-agar flakes dissolve.

2. Meanwhile, bring the pureed fruit to a boil, stirring constantly. Lower heat and continue to cook until thick and most of the water is evaporated, about 20 minutes.

3. Combine the agar-agar mixture with the fruit mixture and allow to sit until firm.

*Note: Agar-agar is a seaweed product available in Asian markets and some health food stores.

CHANTILLY CREAM

1 cup heavy cream
1 teaspoon organic, alcohol-free vanilla extract
1 tablespoon rice syrup

1. Whip the cream with vanilla extract until soft peaks occur.
2. Add the rice syrup and continue to whip until firm.

Variations

1. Omit the rice syrup. Fold 1 cup of fruit filling into the whipped cream.

2. In place of vanilla extract, add 1 teaspoon of either orange, coffee, or coconut extract.

BUTTERCREAM

2 cups (2 sticks) sweet butter, softened
2 egg yolks
5 tablespoons rice syrup
3 teaspoons organic, alcohol-free vanilla extract
1 cup walnuts, chopped (optional)

1. Cream butter and egg yolks until light and fluffy.

2. Blend in the rice syrup and extract and beat until smooth. Fold in walnuts, if desired.

Variations

1. Substitute vanilla with any of the following alcohol-free extracts: coconut, rum, orange, or coffee.

2. Substitute vanilla with ¼ cup of real brewed espresso coffee. Increase butter by 2 tablespoons.

3. Substitute vanilla with ¼ cup orange juice and 1 tablespoon orange zest. Increase butter by 2 tablespoons.

The recipes in this book are the starting point on your journey toward your "perfect ten" recipes. The real magic lies in understanding the *No-Grain Diet* principles so you can continually adjust the program to work for you. Please consult the Resources section of this book for guidance to all that's available to help you start, stabilize, and sustain the *No-Grain* way to health.

In addition, one of the "bonuses" of this book is that the information does not end when you get to the last page. It is designed to be highly interactive with my website, *www.nograindiet.com*, a free re-source designed to make sure you achieve your weight-loss goals. Con-taining extensive and useful health information easily accessed through our search feature, *www.nograindiet.com* is there for your needs. In ad-dition, with other books I look forward to creating, there will be hun-dreds of different recipes from which you can build your "perfect ten." I've designed the *No-Grain Diet* to be a total and ongoing support for your weight-loss and health program. I wish you great success with it!

APPENDIX ONE:
FOOD AND SUPPLEMENTS

My primary focus in treating patients is to use supplements only minimally. High-quality fresh foods are usually sufficient to restore health. Yet obtaining such foods is a major challenge for most Americans. Let me provide you with a few basic guidelines that will help you.

Vegetables

Ideally, it would be great if you could grow your own vegetables. For most of us, this is just not practical or possible. Your next best option is organic vegetables. In late 2002, the U.S. Department of Agriculture finally approved organic standards, and foods that meet these standards will now have a USDA Organic Certification label. But farmers are no different than any other businessmen: if there is not a demand for a product, there will only be limited product. As the demand for organic foods continues, they will become more widely available, but until that time, if you are unable to easily locate organic produce, it is highly likely I will be able to arrange some worthwhile options for you in the near future on *www.nograindiet.com*. Please check that website periodically if you are interested, as I will announce these options as soon as they become available.

However, please, please, please remember: Nonorganic fresh vegetables are better than no vegetables. So if you can't find or afford organic vegetables, please just consume the vegetables at your local grocery store, as those are far preferable to no vegetables at all.

Eggs

Fortunately, high-quality eggs are becoming easier to find in most grocery stores. There are a number of different factors, so let me detail them here.

While organic eggs are preferable, that is not the only consideration. But if the chicken was fed commercial grain exclusively, avoid those eggs since they will be very high in omega-6 fats and low in omega-3 fats.

Now many brands advertise omega-3 eggs, which is a step in the right direction. However, read the carton to determine the source of omega-3. If that's unclear, contact the company to find out. The best source of omega-3 is either flaxseed or fish meal. Canola oil–fed chickens are problematic. Go to *www.nograindiet.com* to find out why I don't recommend canola oil.

Eggs produced from cage-free chickens are another huge plus. You might find these eggs in your local grocery store, or you can encourage the store manager to obtain them.

However, the ultimate eggs are those that you pick up fresh from someone who raises their own chickens. Ideally, the chickens should be fed flaxseeds and also allowed to eat their natural diet from the ground. If you are fortunate enough to locate such eggs, don't refrigerate them, as it degrades the eggs' quality. This is widely understood in South America and Europe.

I recommend raw eggs. This may make some squeamish at first, largely because there's been a lot of misinformation floated around about the danger of raw eggs. Many find them unappetizing, so perhaps I won't convince you to try them. But you should, because many people are deficient in high-quality nutrients that raw eggs contain in abundance, especially high-quality protein and fat. If you follow my guidelines, eggs are much safer than many of the foods you now eat.

Although many people develop food allergies to eggs, I believe this happens because they are cooked. If consumed in their raw state, eggs don't provoke an allergic response. Why? Because heating egg protein changes its chemistry. If you've been unable to tolerate eggs, consider eating them uncooked.

Many people worry about contracting salmonella, a serious infection, with over two-thirds of a million cases annually resulting from eating contaminated eggs. Why, you may wonder, would a competent health care professional recommend eating uncooked eggs? The risk of contracting salmonella from raw eggs is actually quite low. A study by the U.S. Department of Agriculture in early 2002 showed that 2.3 million eggs annually are contaminated with salmonella. However, you need to understand that there are 69 billion eggs produced each year, so only 0.0033 percent of eggs, one in every thirty thousand, is contaminated with salmonella—it's actually quite uncommon.

Nevertheless, to avoid eating a salmonella-contaminated egg, you can learn to decrease your risk of infection. Salmonella infections are usually present only in traditionally raised commercial hens, because only sick chickens lay salmonella-contaminated eggs. High-quality, cage-free, organically fed, omega-3-enhanced chicken eggs, as recommended above, are unlikely to be infected. Still, before you eat eggs, raw or not, I recommend that you thoroughly examine them following these guidelines.

Guidelines for Consuming Fresh High-Quality Eggs

1. Always check the freshness of the egg right before you consume it.

2. If you are uncertain about the freshness of an egg, don't eat it. This is one of the best safeguards against salmonella.

3. If there is a crack in the shell, don't eat it. To check, immerse the egg in a pan of cool, salted water; if it emits a tiny stream of bubbles, the shell is porous, or contains a hole.

4. If your eggs come fresh from a farmer, don't refrigerate them. To judge an egg's freshness, allow it first to come to room temperature for at least one hour.

5. First, check an egg by rolling it across a flat surface. Only consume it if it isn't wobbly.

6. Once you open the egg, if the white is watery, instead of gel-like, if it smells foul, if the yolk is not convex, or if the yolk easily bursts, don't consume it.

How to Start Using Raw Eggs

To begin, start by eating a tiny bit of egg on a daily basis, and then gradually increase the portions. For the first three days, eat only a few drops of raw egg yolk a day. Gradually increase the amount that you consume, in three-day increments. Try half a teaspoon for three days, then one teaspoon, then two teaspoons. Once you're accustomed to that amount, increase it to one raw egg yolk per day and subsequently to two raw egg yolks per day. Eventually, you can easily eat five raw egg yolks daily.

Since fresh raw egg yolk tastes like vanilla, it can be combined with vegetable pulp from your vegetable juice. It can also be combined with avocado. Stir the yolk gently with a fork, because egg protein easily gets damaged on a molecular level.

If you're still worried about salmonella, remember that it's generally a benign and self-limiting illness, especially if you're healthy. However, if you feel sick and have loose stools, the infection can be treated with high-quality probiotics. Take them every thirty minutes until you feel better.

Aren't Raw Egg Whites Unhealthy?

Nutritional dogma advises avoiding raw egg whites because they contain a glycoprotein called avidin that bonds biotin, one of the B vitamins. The concern is that this can lead to a biotin deficiency. The simple solution posed is to cook the egg whites, as this completely deactivates the avidin.

The problem with this approach is that it also completely deactivates nearly every other protein in the egg white. While you will still obtain nutritional benefits from consuming cooked egg whites, from a nutritional perspective it is far better to consume them uncooked.

After my recent studies, it became clear to me that the egg's design carefully compensates for this issue. How does it do that?

It put tons of biotin in the egg yolk. Egg yolks have one of the highest concentrations of biotin found in nature. So it is likely that you will not have a biotin deficiency if you consume the whole raw egg, yolk and white. It is also clear, however, that if you only consume raw egg whites, you are nearly guaranteed to develop a biotin deficiency unless you take a biotin supplement.

There is only a potential problem with using the entire raw egg if you are pregnant. Biotin deficiency is a common concern in pregnancy, and it is possible that consuming whole raw eggs would make it worse.

If you are pregnant, you have two options. The first is to actually measure for a biotin deficiency. This is best done through urinary excretion of 3-hydroxyisovaleric acid (3-HIA), which increases as a result of the decreased activity of the biotin-dependent enzyme methylcrotonyl-CoA carboxylase.

Alternatively, you could take a biotin supplement.

Meat

Truly healthy meat is a particularly challenging food to find. There is clearly a significant and major difference between most commercially raised livestock in this country and—the better choice—livestock that are raised exclusively on grass.

Cattle that are sent to feedlots epitomize the commercial food industry that turns the production of beef into a factory-like process. (For more details of this, please visit *www.nograindiet.com.*)

Once in the feedlot system, they will be exposed to large amounts of corn to fatten them up. These animals were not designed to eat corn, and when their diet is shifted, they tend to get sick, so they receive a variety of immunizations and antibiotics to keep them from dying. They also receive liberal amounts of hormones to maximize their weight gain. This process will virtually shut off their ability to make healthy fat and also change the ratio of the omega-6 to omega-3 fat ratio to one that is far less healthy.

The solution is to consume grass-fed animals. Unfortunately this is not easy to do at this time and can be quite expensive. The most cost-effective solution is to find a farmer who is raising grass-fed cattle and purchase half of a steer. This is generally about three hundred pounds of beef and typically fits quite nicely into one standup freezer. The cost is significantly reduced if you are able to do this.

Please be very careful not to make the mistake I did when I purchased my first half steer. I purchased organic and did not pay attention to what the steer was fed. When I checked that later, I found out that the animal was fed plenty of organic corn. So you are looking for grass-fed cattle only. It is also important to remember that all cattle are grass-fed initially, but prior to fattening them up is when most are fed corn. So be sure and ask to find out the details.

If you are unable to locate grass-fed meats, don't despair, as *www.nograindiet.com* has arranged for a number of distributors to have them available on the site. Grass-fed beef, kosher bison, and two meats I most highly recommend are all available on the site.

Regarding poultry, it is important to recognize that they do require some grains in their diet. However, if they are given grains, you should be certain that they are organic and that they are also not given any pesticides, meat by-products, antibiotics, drugs, growth enhancers, or hormones.

The chart below is also helpful for distinguishing between optimal poultry and free-range that is typically promoted as the best. While free-range is not optimal, it certainly is better than most all commercially raised chickens.

Poultry

Optimal Chickens	Some Free-range and "Natural" Chickens
Raised in small portable pens without bottoms that are moved daily, fed on fresh-planted organic millet, oats, wheat, chicory, and abrassicas, and supplemented with certified organic grains.	"Natural" and free-range meat growers use conventional animal feed that may contain pesticides, toxins, antibiotics, or growth enhancers.
Not debeaked, allowing them to forage easily on pastures.	Free-range birds are commonly debeaked and raised in crowded buildings with access to only barren, fenced yards.
Raising them uses less than 10 percent of the water typically used in factory farming and helps build soil as these birds are grazing and composting.	Free-range and "Natural" birds raised in large factory-farmed buildings excessively waste "potable water" and pollute aquifers with runoff from waste piles.

(continued)

Optimal Chickens	Some Free-range and "Natural" Chickens
Moved daily over fields of fresh greens, allowing fresh air and sunshine into the pens and eliminating any contamination with pathogens and parasites.	Free-range and "Natural" chickens raised in large factory-farmed buildings allow for contamination with parasites and pathogens with buildup of fecal matter and poor ventilation.

Finding the Best Meats

The three meats I most highly recommend for their exceptional nutritional value, along with great taste, are bison (also known as buffalo), ostrich, and grass-fed beef.

Bison has rapidly found its way onto the menu of many five-star restaurants and onto the meat rack of select grocery stores in the U.S. over the past decade. It tends to be even sweeter and more tender than beef—many people claim that bison is simply the best-tasting meat they've ever had.

Both bison and ostrich also have similar protein levels to beef. The best news, though, is that they are lower in calories, cholesterol, and fat than beef, pork, and even skinless turkey and chicken!

When choosing bison, please ensure they have been raised as free-range animals in an ecologically sound and humane manner, with vegetation as their prime forage. Also make sure their label notes that they were raised without antibiotics, hormones, or steroids.

As grain is a natural part of any bird's diet, you will not likely find ostrich that haven't consumed some grain. If you have gone completely *No-Grain*, take this into consideration; if you are only consuming grains in moderation, the better brands of ostrich, like Blackwing, only feed their birds about 20 percent grains.

You can find bison at grocery stores and health food stores in many parts of the country, such as the Whole Foods Market chain. You can also contact the National Bison Association in Denver, Colorado, or go to their website at *www.bisoncentral.com*, for a list of retail and mail-order stores in the U.S. and Canada. Both ostrich and bison are also offered at *www.nograindiet.com* (including Glatt Kosher bison).

For those following a diet entirely exclusive of grains, another out-standing meat is grass-fed beef. This is precisely what its name says—cattle allowed to feed in their natural manner, entirely upon the grasses on a range. Almost all the beef you buy at the grocery store or in restaurants is from cattle who have been fed a diet high in grains to fat-ten them up quickly—problem is, its effects are very similar in people. For this reason—not to mention the effects of antibiotics, hormones, and other additives—pay close attention to the diet of your meat.

Grass-fed beef is naturally lean, so if you are used to eating the fat-test parts of grain-fed beef, it will take some getting used to, but the taste is still excellent. Grass-fed beef, meanwhile, is far superior to grain-fed beef in terms of nutrition. Unlike grain-fed beef, grass-fed is an outstanding source of omega-3 fats—the "good fat" that most Americans are dangerously deficient in. It is high in beta-carotene and con-tains 400 percent more of vitamins A and E than grain-fed beef. Finally, unlike "normal" beef, grass-fed is also high in conjugated linoleic acid, which research has shown actually helps prevent those who have lost weight from regaining those pounds.

The best way to purchase grass-fed beef is probably the most incon-venient—from a local rancher raising such beef. In relation to organic farming, this is becoming more popular, though people living in and around major cities will obviously find it impractical. Still, if you can find such a source, and you don't mind taking a weekend drive, the per-pound price you pay will be much lower than what you'll pay in any store. I have, in fact, occasionally purchased an entire side of beef in this manner. The savings in cost far outweighed the hassles of stor-ing the meat in my freezer, plus I was spared having to buy meat for some time. Of course, this simply won't be practical for many.

So, just as with bison, check your local grocery store or health food store for grass-fed beef. More and more stores are stocking it; as always, though, read the label carefully to ensure it is entirely grass-fed. It is also available online at *www.nograindiet.com* and a variety of other sites (a simple search for the term at Google or another search engine will yield a number of worthwhile results).

Juicers

If you are new to juicing, consider starting with an inexpensive centrifugal juicer. Krups juicers are a good starting point in this category, and you can easily find them at Crate and Barrel and other stores.

Once you are convinced that you will be doing vegetable juicing long-term, consider investing in a higher-quality juicer that makes far less noise and is easier and quicker to clean up. I did an extensive evaluation of different juicers (comparison available on *www.nograindiet. com*) and concluded that single-geared juicers are the best value. Some of these can get quite pricey, but I use the Omega 8001 that retails for around $300 but is widely available on the Internet for about $40 less than that.

Supplements

With all supplements pay careful attention to ensure high quality, which is why I highly recommend purchasing them from your local health food store. They are generally quite knowledgeable about the different brands and potencies, and can recognize "spoiled" or otherwise undesirable aspects of the supplements. If you have any problems with the supplements, they usually allow you to return them, as well.

If you cannot find a supplement at your health food store, use the Internet to locate a reputable source. Google is an excellent search engine to start with, but when you reach a site, try to read as much as you can about that site to find out who runs it and why they are pushing a particular brand. At *www.nograindiet.com*, I only recommend products that I truly believe in. I specifically recommend Carlson's brand fish oil and cod liver oil, for instance, while advising against certain other fish oil brands. I don't accept advertising money, so my decisions are based on medical opinion, not finances. It may take a little research on your part, but it is not hard to detect those sites whose "recommendations" were purchased in one way or another. Avoid them.

APPENDIX TWO: EFT

Guidelines for Those Seeking a Therapist

by Dr. Patricia Carrington
http://www.eftsupport.com/guideline_therapists.htm

Searching for a suitable therapist is similar to searching for an appropriate physician, dentist, attorney, or any other professional who meets your needs. It is not always easy to discover the right person and there are no blanket rules for doing so. However, if you keep the following points in mind this should make the process easier and more satisfactory for you.

Initial Contact with Therapist

You will usually want to speak with the therapist or coach (at least briefly) before making an appointment to start working with him or her. During this first contact you can find out certain facts about their background, training, fees, and details of their practice that are important for you to know.

If the therapist has a website, many of these details are usually given there, but you will still want to talk with that person or at least make contact by email because you will need to know more about them than facts alone can supply.

Your initial contact with a prospective therapist will give you an idea of whether this is a perceptive, caring person with whom you could feel comfortable talking and sharing your personal problems. Professional degrees alone, while essential if you have serious emotional problems, do not tell you whether or not this person will be an effective therapist for you.

Only you can determine this, and on a "gut level." If you respond positively to this therapist during the initial contact and feel that they are a person whom you can probably trust, then you can feel confident in scheduling a session.

An initial "trial" (paid for) session with the therapist you have selected is an excellent way to determine whether they are indeed right for you, and you are entirely within your rights to let the therapist know that you want to schedule such a trial session.

You will notice that a number of the therapists on Gary Craig's list of EFT-trained practitioners offer a free twenty-minute exploratory discussion by telephone to help you decide this. That can be very useful if available; however, a number of therapists do not do this, and this fact does not necessarily make them less competent or useful—they may simply be too heavily booked to be able to offer that free time.

Therefore, the best plan is to schedule a trial paid session with them and see how that works out. Even if you decide not to work with that therapist in the future, in this session you may well accomplish something of genuine value, particularly since the therapist is working with such a rapid technique as EFT.

What to Look for in Terms of Training

Most qualified practitioners in the field of mental health (but not necessarily in allied health fields) hold graduate degrees such as a Ph.D. (usually these are psychologists), LCSW (licensed clinical social worker), or M.D. (medical doctor, usually one specializing in psychiatry). These and similar degrees indicate that these people have undergone an internship and supervised training in their field of specialty.

Most professionals will also be licensed by a recognized professional licensing board and belong to one or more professional associations. Don't hesitate to inquire about licensing (it will be necessary if you seek insurance reimbursement) and other aspects of their background. While professional licensing ensures that the therapist has completed the requisite training and internships in their field of specialty, it does not give you any information about their competency. "Therapeutic touch" is not conferred by degrees or licenses; many who have it may have no such credentials.

You will notice, for example, that there are EFT practitioners on the list who do not qualify for professional licensing, yet some of them are brilliant natural clinicians and "healers" who may be extremely helpful to you, providing you do not have a recognized emotional disturbance that requires treatment by a licensed mental health practitioner.

In this vein, it is significant to note that the founder of EFT, Gary Craig, does not have a professional license in the field of mental health (he is a personal performance coach, minister, and engineer), but he has a rare ability to assist people when using EFT and is a prime example of therapeutic gifts that far exceed any formal training. (*Note:* Gary Craig is not presently available for individual therapy due to his many commitments.)

Finding an EFT Practitioner or Therapist (http://www.eftsupport.com/find_therapist.htm)

Note: If you have an especially traumatic, complex, or deep-seated issue to deal with, it is advisable to work with EFT, as with any other stress management technique, under the supervision of a qualified mental health professional.

Locating a therapist, counselor, coach, or other health care professional who will meet your personal needs always means searching, but it is well worth the effort when you find the right one.

Strengths and Limitations of the Lists

Each EFT practitioner who is on Gary Craig's list, in addition to submitting a description of his or her work, also fills out a standardized questionnaire, and their responses to the questions asked are given with each entry, allowing you to make somewhat of a comparison between the practitioners' backgrounds.

Because the persons included on these lists volunteered to be listed on them, the lists are not exhaustive and you may find that some highly qualified EFT-trained therapists are not represented on them. However, you will get some very useful leads from them nevertheless, and if you are seeking an EFT therapist you may well want to consult them. Here are some pointers to keep in mind if you do so:

Indications of Practitioner Competency

Neither of these lists provide information about the competency of the practitioners they list; they might be compared to the yellow pages of a telephone book which steer you to individuals who offer the services you are seeking, but does not evaluate them. It is therefore up to you to explore the suitability of any particular practitioner for your own needs.

Format

Both lists group practitioners by state (in the U.S.) and by country elsewhere, a very useful device if you are seeking in-office treatment. However, there is another option, which many people find extremely useful, which is EFT sessions by telephone.

Many practitioners and their clients consider EFT telephone therapy to be just as effective as in-office therapy, and in some cases it may even be preferred. The reasons EFT phone therapy is so popular are:

Concentration on the issue at hand may actually be greater during a telephone session than in an office visit because visual distractions that occur in an office setting are entirely absent.

Phone sessions provide special benefits in terms of saved time and cost of traveling, and provide for much greater flexibility of scheduling.

Looking for a therapist who can work with you by phone allows you to select from a much wider list of EFT therapists in many different locations, including some of the acknowledged leaders in the field—a much more comprehensive selection than can be found in any single vicinity.

Fees to Expect

The cost of EFT-oriented psychotherapy or counseling is exactly the same as that of any other form of psychotherapy, counseling, personal performance coaching, or any other service by health practitioners who are specially trained in their area. Fees vary widely from practitioner to practitioner depending upon the practitioner's credentials and their standing in their own specialty area, as well as their expertise in EFT.

Telephone sessions are charged for at the same hourly rate as in-office visits because both demand an equal amount of time, skill, and commitment on the part of the therapist. You cannot expect a special financial arrangement because you opt for a phone appointment.

Exactly what will you pay? In general, fees per session will range from $60 to $175, with the average fee falling somewhere in the $80 to $125 range. While these may be the customary fees for the professional services you are seeking, bear in mind that therapy using EFT is often more rapid than a conventional approach and therefore may be more cost effective in the long run.

However, ongoing treatment over time is often required for deeper issues, so this should be planned for accordingly. Insurance reimbursement may or may not be obtainable for EFT-oriented psychotherapy, depending on the professional requirements and geographical constraints of your insurance carrier.

Practitioner's Expertise in EFT

When evaluating EFT practitioners, in addition to assessing their professional qualifications, we suggest you pay careful attention to how much experience each practitioner has had with EFT, what their training has been in this method, approximately how many people they have treated with EFT, and other details indicating the extent of their familiarity with this technique.

Sometimes you can judge the skill with which a practitioner applies EFT by reading some of the EFT Case Histories on Gary Craig's website, *www.emofree.com*. In that section you will find accounts written by therapists about their EFT work with clients.

This may help you judge certain therapists' competence in administering EFT, although many a highly skilled practitioner of EFT has not had the opportunity to contribute to Gary's email lists and may not, therefore, have their work represented on his site. Reading over the reports of those practitioners posted on that site, however, should give you an idea of how sensitive these therapists are to their clients' problems and how creative they are in applying EFT.

APPENDIX THREE: MEDICAL TESTS

Thyroid Testing

Over 15 million Americans are unaware of and undiagnosed for their thyroid conditions. Are you one of them? If you are a pregnant woman and you have a low thyroid, your child's IQ will be affected. Researchers have also shown that if you an elderly woman with thyroid problems you will have an increased risk of heart disease.

If Your Doctor Can't Interpret Your Tests Properly

The big myth that persists regarding thyroid diagnosis is that an elevated TSH (thyroid stimulating hormone) level is always required before a diagnosis of hypothyroidism (underactive thyroid) can be made. Normally, the pituitary gland will secrete TSH in response to a low thyroid hormone level. Thus an elevated TSH level would typically suggest an underactive thyroid.

Thyroid function tests have always presented doctors with difficulties in their interpretation. Laboratory testing is often misleading due to the complexity and inherent shortcomings of the tests themselves. Many doctors do not having an adequate understanding of what the test results mean and will often make incorrect assumptions based on them, or interpret them too strictly. A narrow interpretation of thyroid function testing leads to many people not being treated for subclinical hypothyroidism.

Old Laboratory Tests Unreliable

Most older thyroid function panels include the following:

Total T4

T3Uptake

Free Thyroxine Index (FTI)

These tests are unreliable as gauges of thyroid function. The most common traditional way to diagnose hypothyroidism is with a TSH that is elevated beyond the normal reference range. For most labs, this is about 4.0 to 4.5. This is thought to reflect the pituitary's sensing of inadequate thyroid hormone levels in the blood, which would be consistent with hypothyroidism. There is no question that this will diagnose hypothyroidism, but it is far too insensitive a measure, and the vast majority of patients who have hypothyroidism will be missed.

Basal Body Temperature

Basal body temperature was popularized by the late Broda Barnes, M.D. He found clinical symptoms and body temperature to be more reliable gauges than the standard laboratory tests. However, there are problems with using body temperature:

Sleeping under electric blankets or on water beds falsely raises temperature.

A sensitive and accurate thermometer is required.

Checking it is inconvenient, and many people will not do it (poor compliance).

New and More Accurate Way to Check for Hypothyroidism

A revised method of diagnosing and treating hypothyroidism seems superior to the temperature regulation method promoted by Broda

Barnes and many natural medicine physicians. Most patients continue to have classic hypothyroid symptoms because excessive reliance is placed on the TSH. This test is a highly accurate measure of TSH but not of the height of thyroid hormone levels.

New Range for TSH to Diagnose Hypothyroidism

The basic problem that traditional medicine has with diagnosing hypothyroidism is that the so-called "normal range" of TSH is far too high. Many patients with TSHs of greater than 2.0 (not 4.5) have classic symptoms and signs of hypothyroidism (see below). If your TSH is above 3.0, there is a strong chance your thyroid gland is not working properly.

Free Thyroid Hormone Levels

One can also use the Free T3 and Free T4 with TSH levels to help one identify how well the thyroid gland is working. Free T3 and Free T4 levels are the only accurate measure of the actual active thyroid hormone levels in the blood. When free hormone levels are tested, it is relatively common to find the Free T4 and Free T3 hormone levels below normal when TSH is in its normal range, even in the low end of its normal range. When patients with these lab values are treated, one typically finds tremendous improvement in the patient, and a reduction of the classic hypothyroid symptoms.

Secondary or Tertiary Hypothyroidism

There are a significant number of individuals who have a TSH even below the new 2.0 reference range but their Free T3 (and possibly the Free T4 as well) will be below normal. These are cases of secondary or tertiary hypothyroidism, so TSH alone is not an accurate test of all forms of hypothyroidism, only primary hypothyroidism.

Symptoms of Low Thyroid

You can also use the following symptoms as a sensitive measure of how well your thyroid gland is working.

Fatigue

Skin that is dry, cold, rough, and scaly

Hair that is coarse, brittle, and grows slowly or may fall out excessively

Sensitivity to cold, with feelings of being chilly in rooms of normal temperature

Difficulty sweating, and decreased or even absent perspiration during heavy exercise and hot weather

Constipation that is resistant to magnesium supplementation and other mild laxatives

Difficulty in losing weight despite rigid adherence to a low-grain diet (especially in women)

Depression and muscle weakness

Natural Thyroid Treatment

However, it is important to note that even if your thyroid gland isn't working, in my experience it is likely related to emotional stresses that impair the adrenal gland. Once the adrenal gland becomes impaired, the thyroid seeks to compensate and eventually it too starts to fail.

Treating the thyroid or adrenal with hormone supplements does not address the foundation of the problem. The danger of using thyroid hormones is that your thyroid gland tends to permanently shut down after 3 to 5 years on the hormones, and it will be nearly impossible to wean yourself off of them.

So rather than condemning a person to thyroid hormones their entire life, in my practice I seek to address the underlying emotional stressors. I typically send them to one of the therapists in my office that use EFT treatments, to help them resolve the physical effects of stress on their adrenal and thyroid glands, and we are frequently able to help resolve the problem.

Additionally, one can use iodide and selenium supplements to further help the thyroid gland do its work. If you have profound thyroid dysfunction or the natural treatments have not worked, then you are a candidate for thyroid hormone replacement.

Should You Use Synthetic Hormones?

The traditional approach is to use synthetic hormones like Synthroid/Levoxyl/Levothroid (levothyroxine). These products only contain T4 hormone; they have no T3. When patients attempt to ask their physicians for the natural hormone, they are usually ridiculed and made to feel stupid that they would request an inferior hormone product. The common argument the physicians give is that the synthetic provides steadier hormone levels. What the doctors tend to overlook is that the vast majority of people cannot convert the T4 in them to the active form of thyroid, which is T3. This is easy to confirm by measuring the free hormone levels, but virtually none of the doctors use these tests.

Armour Thyroid—The Natural Alternative

When one has low T3 levels, which are typical with synthetic hormone use, the brain does not work properly. It is important to use a preparation that contains both T3 and T4 because T3 does 90 percent of the work of the thyroid in the body. So one should use a combination of T4 and T3, which compensates for the inability to convert T4 to T3. Armour Thyroid is desiccated thyroid and has both T3 and T4.

A 1999 study published in one of the most prestigious medical journals in the world, the *New England Journal of Medicine,* showed that a natural hormone product, such as Armour, was far better at controlling the brain problems commonly found in hypothyroidism. Nearly all natural medicine doctors tend to use Armour Thyroid, which is a mixture of mono- and di-iodothryonine and T3 and T4, the entire range of thyroid hormones.

Armour Thyroid Dosing—*Twice* a Day

The most common starting dose for patients with hypothyroidism is 90 mg of Armour Thyroid that is cut in half with a razor blade, with half taken after breakfast and the other half after dinner. Taking it after meals also helps to reduce volatility of the blood-level of T3. If the patient has any problem breaking or cutting the pill, a pill-cutter can be purchased at the pharmacy. The TSH, Free T3, and Free T4 tests are then repeated in one month and the dose is adjusted.

Taking the Armour Thyroid twice a day overcomes traditional medicine's major objection and resistance to using natural thyroid preparations—variability in its blood-levels. Most doctors using Armour Thyroid are not aware that Armour Thyroid should be used twice daily and *not* once a day. The major reason is that the T3 component has such a short half-life and needs to be taken twice daily to achieve consistent blood levels.

Dose Adjustments with Lab Monitoring

Once a patient is on hormone replacement, the dose can be increased until the TSH falls below 0.4. Then one needs to optimize the two thyroid hormones by testing the Free T4 and Free T3 levels. They should be above the median (middle) but below the upper end of the normal laboratory reference range. The goal for healthy young adults would be to have numbers close to the upper part of the range, and for cardiac and/or elderly patients, the numbers should be in the middle range.

The Free T3 and Free T4 levels should be checked every four weeks, and the hormone therapy readjusted until the FT3 and FT4 levels are in the therapeutic range described. Once a therapeutic range is achieved, the levels should be checked at least once a year. A small number of large, overweight, thyroid-resistant women may need 6 to 8 grains of Armour Thyroid or the equivalent of thyroxine per day (counting 0.1 mg of T4 as 1 grain of Armour Thyroid).

Those people who are already on once daily Armour thyroid should split the dose and take half after breakfast and half after dinner. Since the only change will be in the FT3 level, which has a short half-life, the serum FT4 and FT3 levels (and TSH, if indicated) can be measured forty-eight to seventy-two hours after beginning to split the doses if the patient was on the hormone for four to six weeks before the splitting began. This is because the Free T4 hormone is the one that takes a number of weeks to build up to its steady-state serum level.

Symptoms of Excessive Thyroid Hormone

These are frequently only temporary during the treatment adaptation stage. However, if they persist, you will certainly want to lower your dose of thyroid hormones. The symptoms may include:

Palpitations

Nervousness

Feeling hot and sweaty

Rapid weight loss

Fine tremor

Clammy skin

What to Do If You Cannot Tolerate Armour Thyroid or Want to Continue Synthetic Hormones

My experience is that well over 90 percent of people do much better on Armour Thyroid. However, there are a small number of people who do not tolerate it. Cytomel, which is T3 only, can be used in combination with one of the T4-only synthetic preparations mentioned above. It is important to recognize that T3 should be taken twice daily due to its shorter half-life. This is typically after breakfast and supper because that makes it easier to remember.

If you are currently taking Synthroid (thyroxine), your Free T4 level is probably at or above the high end of its normal range and your Free T3 level is likely below. In this situation, one may then add 5 to 12.5 mcg Cytomel (pure T3) after breakfast and supper daily, rather than Armour Thyroid or Thyrolar (synthetic T4/T3 combo). With one or two doses daily, one can then optimize both the T4 and T3 levels, with whatever thyroid preparation is required. This is not possible in most hypothyroid patients with T4-only preparations.

REFERENCES

Chapter One

Flegal, K.M., M.D. Carroll, C.L. Ogden, et al. "Prevalence and trends in obesity among US adults, 1999–2000." *Journal of the American Medical Association*, October 9, 2002; 288:1723–1727.
http://www.ncbi.nlm.nih.gov/entrez/query.fcgi?cmd=Retrieve&db=PubMed&list=_uid s=12365955&dopt=Abstract

Pollan, Michael. "Power Steer." *New York Times Magazine*, March 31, 2002.
http://www.nytimes.com/2002/03/31/magazine/31BEEF.html?pagewanted=all& position-top

Taubes, Gary. "What If It's All Been a Big Fat Lie?" *New York Times Magazine*, July 7, 2002.
http://www.nytimes.com/2002/07/07/magazine/07FAT.html?ex=1027146737&ei=1 &en=a6afd75e34e60e3a

Chapter Two

Abbasi, F., B.W. Brown, Jr., C. Lamendola, et al. "Relationship between obesity, insulin resistance, and coronary heart disease risk." *Journal of the American College Cardiology,* September 4, 2002; 40(5): 937–943.
http://www.ncbi.nlm.nih.gov/entrez/query.fcgi?cmd=Retrieve&db=PubMed&list=_uid s=12225719&dopt=Abstract

Abdulkarim, A.S., L.J. Burgart, J. See. "Etiology of nonresponsive celiac disease: results of a systematic approach." *American Journal of Gastroenterology*, August 2002; 97(8): 2016–2021.

http://www.ncbi.nlm.nih.gov/entrez/query.fcgi?cmd=Retrieve&db=PubMed&list=_uid s=12190170&dopt=Abstract

Andersen, R.E., C.J. Crespo, S.J. Bartlett, et al. "Relationship of physical activity and television watching with body weight and level of fatness among children: results from the Third National Health and Nutrition Examination Survey." *JAMA*, March 25, 1998; 279(12): 938–942.
http://www.ncbi.nlm.nih.gov/entrez/query.fcgi?cmd=Retrieve&db=PubMed&list=_uid s=9544768&dopt=Abstract

Anderson, G.H., N.L. Catherine, D.M. Woodend, et al. "Inverse association between the effect of carbohydrates on blood glucose and subsequent short-term food intake in young men." *American Journal of Clinical Nutrition*, November 2002; 76(5):1023–1030.
http://www.ncbi.nlm.nih.gov/entrez/query.fcgi?cmd=Retrieve&db=PubMed&list=_uid s=12399274&dopt=Abstract

Augustin, L.S., S. Franceschi, D.J. Jenkins, et al. "Glycemic index in chronic disease: a review." *European Journal Clinical Nutrition*. November 2002; 56(11): 1049–1071.
http://www.ncbi.nlm.nih.gov/entrez/query.fcgi?cmd=Retrieve&db=PubMed&list=_uid s=12428171&dopt=Abstract

Brand-Miller, J.C., S.H. Holt, D.B. Pawlak, J. McMillan. "Glycemic index and obesity." *American Journal Clinical Nutrition*, July 2002; 76(1):281S–285S.
http://www.ncbi.nlm.nih.gov/entrez/query.fcgi?cmd=Retrieve&db=PubMed&list=_uid s=12081852&dopt=Abstract

Castelli, W.P. "Concerning the possibility of a nut . . ." *Archive Internal Medicine*, July 1992; 152(7):1371–1372.
http://www.ncbi.nlm.nih.gov/entrez/query.fcgi?cmd=Retrieve&db=PubMed&list=_uid s=1303626&dopt=Abstract

Collin, P., K. Kaukinen, M. Valimaki, J. Salmi. "Endocrinological disorders and celiac disease." *Endocrinology Review*, August 2002; 23(4):464–483.
http://www.ncbi.nlm.nih.gov/entrez/query.fcgi?cmd=Retrieve&db=PubMed&list=_uid s=12202461&dopt=Abstract

Cordain, L., S.B. Eaton, J. Brand-Miller, et al. "An evolutionary analysis of the aetiology and pathogenesis of juvenile-onset myopia." *Acta Ophthalmol Scand*, April 2002; 80(2):125–135.
http://www.ncbi.nlm.nih.gov/entrez/query.fcgi?cmd=Retrieve&db=PubMed&list=_uid s=11952477&dopt=Abstract

Cordain, L., S.B. Eaton, J.B. Miller, et al. "The paradoxical nature of hunter-gatherer diets: meat-based, yet non-atherogenic." *European Journal of Clinical Nutrition*, March 2002; 56 Suppl 1:S42–S52.
http://www.ncbi.nlm.nih.gov/entrez/query.fcgi?cmd=Retrieve&db=PubMed&list=_uids=11965522&dopt=Abstract

Cordain, L., J.B. Miller, S.B. Eaton, et al. "Macronutrient estimations in hunter-gatherer diets." *American Journal of Clinical Nutrition,* December 2000; 72(6): 1589–1592.
http://www.ajcn.org/cgi/content/full/72/6/1589

Cordain, L., B.A. Watkins, G.L. Florant, et al. "Fatty acid analysis of wild ruminant tissues: evolutionary implications for reducing diet-related chronic disease." *European Journal of Clinical Nutrition*, March 2002; 56(3):181–191.
http://www.ncbi.nlm.nih.gov/entrez/query.fcgi?cmd=Retrieve&db=PubMed&list=_uids=11960292&dopt=Abstract

Cordain, L., S. Lindeberg, M. Hurtado, et al. "Acne vulgaris: a disease of Western civilization." *Arch Dermatol,* December 2002; 138(12):1584–1590.
http://www.ncbi.nlm.nih.gov/entrez/query.fcgi?cmd=Retrieve&db=PubMed&list=_uids=12472346&dopt=Abstract

Eaton, S.B., L. Cordain, S. Lindeberg. "Evolutionary health promotion: a consideration of common counterarguments." *Preventive Medicine*, February 2002; 34(2):119–123.
http://www.ncbi.nlm.nih.gov/entrez/query.fcgi?cmd=Retrieve&db=PubMed&list=_uids=11817904&dopt=Abstract

Eaton, S.B., B.I. Strassman, Nesse, et al. "Evolutionary health promotion." *Preventive Medicine,* February 2002; 34(2):109–118.
http://www.ncbi.nlm.nih.gov/entrez/query.fcgi?cmd=Retrieve&db=PubMed&list=_uids=11817903&dopt=Abstract

Eaton, S.B., L. Cordain, S.B. Eaton. "An evolutionary foundation for health promotion." *World Review Nutrition Diet,* 2001; 90:5–12.
http://www.ncbi.nlm.nih.gov/entrez/query.fcgi?cmd=Retrieve&db=PubMed&list=_uids=11545045&dopt=Abstract

Ebbeling, C.B., D.B. Pawlak, D.S. Ludwig. "Childhood obesity: public-health crisis, common sense cure." *Lancet,* August 10, 2002; 360(9331):473–482.
http://www.ncbi.nlm.nih.gov/entrez/query.fcgi?cmd=Retrieve&db=PubMed&list=_uids=12241736&dopt=Abstract

Eisenstein, J., S.B. Roberts, G. Dallal, et al. "High-protein weight-loss diets: are they safe and do they work? A review of the experimental and epidemiologic data." *Nutrition Reviews,* July 2002; 60(7 Pt 1):189–200.
http://www.ncbi.nlm.nih.gov/entrez/query.fcgi?cmd=Retrieve&db=PubMed&list=_uid s=12144197&dopt=Abstract

Enig, M.G. "Know Your Fats," 114–115; (b) M.G. Enig. "Lauric oils as antimicrobial agents: theory of effect, scientific rationale, and dietary application as adjunct nutritional support for HIV-infected individuals," in *Nutrients and Foods in AIDS,* R.R. Watson, editor, (CRC Press; FL.), 1999, 81–97.

Febbraio, M.A., J. Keenan, D.J. Angus, et al. "Pre-exercise carbohydrate ingestion, glucose kinetics, and muscle glycogen use: effect of the glycemic index." *Journal of Applied Physiology,* 2000; 89:1845–1851.
http://www.ncbi.nlm.nih.gov/entrez/query.fcgi?cmd=Retrieve&db=PubMed&list=_uid s=11053335&dopt=Abstract

Flegal, K.M., M.D. Carroll. C.L. Ogden. "Prevalence and Trends in Obesity Among US Adults, 1999–2000." *JAMA,* October 9, 2002; 288(14):1723–1727.
http://www.ncbi.nlm.nih.gov/entrez/query.fcgi?cmd=Retrieve&db=PubMed&list=_uid s=12365955&dopt=Abstract

Fleming, D.J., K.L. Tucker, P.F. Jacques, et al. "Dietary factors associated with the risk of high iron stores in the elderly Framingham Heart Study cohort." *American Journal of Clinical Nutrition,* December 2002; 76(6):1189–1190.
http://www.ncbi.nlm.nih.gov/entrez/query.fcgi?cmd=Retrieve&db=PubMed&list=_uid s=12450906&dopt=Abstract

Ghezzi, A., M. Zaffaroni. "Neurological manifestations of gastrointestinal disorders, with particular reference to the differential diagnosis of multiple sclerosis." *Neurological Science,* November 2001; 22 Suppl 2:S117–S122.
http://www.ncbi.nlm.nih.gov/entrez/query.fcgi?cmd=Retrieve&db=PubMed&list=_uid s=11794474&dopt=Abstract

Grundy, S.M. "Obesity, metabolic syndrome, and coronary atherosclerosis." *Circulation,* June 11, 2002; 105(23):2696–2698.
http://www.ncbi.nlm.nih.gov/entrez/query.fcgi?cmd=Retrieve&db=PubMed&list=_uid s=12057978&cular reference to

Grundy, S. "The Optimal ratio of fat to carbohydrate in the diet." *Annual Review of Nutrition;* 1999; 19:325–341.
http://www.ncbi.nlm.nih.gov/entrez/query.fcgi?cmd=Retrieve&db=PubMed&list=_uid s=10448527&dopt=Abstract

Hadjivassiliou, M., R.A. Grunewald, G.A. Davies-Jones. "Gluten sensitivity as a neurological illness." *Journal of Neurology, Neurosurgery and Psychiatry*, May 2002; 72(5):560–563.
http://www.ncbi.nlm.nih.gov/entrez/query.fcgi?cmd=Retrieve&db=PubMed&list=_uid s=11971034&dopt=Abstract

Hasler, W.L. "Celiac sprue as a possible cause of symptoms in presumed irritable bowel syndrome." *Gastroenterology*, June 2002; 122(7):2086-2–87.
http://www.ncbi.nlm.nih.gov/entrez/query.fcgi?cmd=Retrieve&db=PubMed&list=_uid s=12078669&dopt=Abstract

Heaney, R.P. "Nutritional factors in osteoporosis." *Annual Review Nutrition*, 1993; 13:287–316.
http://www.ncbi.nlm.nih.gov/entrez/query.fcgi?cmd=Retrieve&db=PubMed&list=_uid s=8369148&dopt=Abstract

Heath, R.J., S.W. White, C.O. Rock. "Inhibitors of fatty acid synthesis as antimicrobial chemotherapeutics." *Applied Microbiological Biotechnology*, May 2002; 58(6):695–703.
http://www.ncbi.nlm.nih.gov/entrez/query.fcgi?cmd=Retrieve&db=PubMed&list=_uid s=12021787&dopt=Abstract

Howarth, N.C., E. Saltzman, S.B. Roberts. "Dietary fiber and weight regulation." *Nutrition Reviews*, May 2001; 59(5):129–139.
http://www.ncbi.nlm.nih.gov/entrez/query.fcgi?cmd=Retrieve&db=PubMed&list=_uid s=11396693&dopt=Abstract

Leeds, A.R. "Glycemic index and heart disease." *American Journal Clinical Nutrition*, July 2002; 76(1):286S–289S.
http://www.ncbi.nlm.nih.gov/entrez/query.fcgi?cmd=Retrieve&db=PubMed&list=_uid s=12081853&dopt=Abstract

Liu, S., W.C. Willett. "Dietary glycemic load and atherothrombotic risk." *Current Atherosclerosis Report*, November 2002; 4(6):454–461.
http://www.ncbi.nlm.nih.gov/entrez/query.fcgi?cmd=Retrieve&db=PubMed&list=_uid s=12361493&dopt=Abstract

Hu, F.B., J.E. Manson, M.J. Stampfer, et al. "Diet, lifestyle, and the risk of type 2 diabetes mellitus in women." *New England Journal of Medicine*, September 13, 2001; 345(11):790–797.
http://www.ncbi.nlm.nih.gov/entrez/query.fcgi?cmd=Retrieve&db=PubMed&list=_uid s=11556298&dopt=Abstract

Jenkins, D.J., C.W. Kendall, L.S. Augustin, et al. "Glycemic index: overview of implications in health and disease." *American Journal of Clinical Nutrition*, July 2002; 76(1):266S–2673S.
http://www.ncbi.nlm.nih.gov/entrez/query.fcgi?cmd=Retrieve&db=PubMed&list=_uids=12081850&dopt=Abstract

Kantor, L.S., et al. "Choose a Variety of Grains Daily, Especially Whole Grains: A challenge for consumers." *The Journal of Nutrition*, Vol. 131, No. 2S-I, February 2001: 473S–486S.
http://www.nutrition.org/cgi/reprint/131/2/473S.pdf

Ludwig, D.S. "Dietary glycemic index and obesity." *Journal of Nutrition*, 2000; 130(suppl):280S–283S.
http://www.ncbi.nlm.nih.gov/entrez/query.fcgi?cmd=Retrieve&db=PubMed&list=_uids=11480757&dopt=Abstract

Ludwig, D.S. "The glycemic index: physiological mechanisms relating to obesity, diabetes, and cardiovascular disease." *JAMA*, May 8, 2002; 287(18): 2414–2423.
http://www.ncbi.nlm.nih.gov/entrez/query.fcgi?cmd=Retrieve&db=PubMed&list=_uids=11988062&dopt=Abstract

Ludwig, D.S., J.A. Majzoub, A. Al-Zahrani, et al. "High glycemic index foods, overeating, and obesity." *Pediatrics*, March 1999; 103(3):E26.
http://www.ncbi.nlm.nih.gov/entrez/query.fcgi?cmd=Retrieve&db=PubMed&list=_uids=10049982&dopt=Abstract

McCarty, M.F. "The origins of western obesity: a role for animal protein?" *Medical Hypotheses*, March 2000; 54(3):488–494.
http://www.ncbi.nlm.nih.gov/entrez/query.fcgi?cmd=Retrieve&db=PubMed&list=_uids=10783494&dopt=Abstract

Mainardi, E., A. Montanelli, M. Dotti, et al. "Thyroid-related autoantibodies and celiac disease: a role for a gluten-free diet?" *Journal of Clinical Gastroenterology*, September 2002; 35(3):245–248.
http://www.ncbi.nlm.nih.gov/entrez/query.fcgi?cmd=Retrieve&db=PubMed&list=_uids=12192201&dopt=Abstract

Mercola, J.M. "Low-Fat Diets Will Increase, Not Decrease, Triglycerides: Some Vegetable Alternatives." *Can Medical Journal*, January 2003.

Pi-Sunyer, F.X. "Glycemic index and disease." *American Journal Clinical Nutrition*, July 2002; 76(1):290S–298S.
http://www.ncbi.nlm.nih.gov/entrez/query.fcgi?cmd=Retrieve&db=PubMed&list=_uids=12081854&dopt=Abstract

Popat, S., S. Bevan, C.P. Braegger, et al. "Genome screening of coeliac disease." *Journal of Medical Genetics,* May 2002; 39(5):328–331.
http://www.ncbi.nlm.nih.gov/entrez/query.fcgi?cmd=Retrieve&db=PubMed&list=_uid s=12011149&dopt=Abstract

Ramakrishnan, U., E. Kuklina A.D. Stein. "Iron stores and cardiovascular disease risk factors in women of reproductive age in the United States." *American Journal of Clinical Nutrition,* December 2002; 76(6):1256–1260.
http://www.ncbi.nlm.nih.gov/entrez/query.fcgi?cmd=Retrieve&db=PubMed&list=_uid s=12450891&dopt=Abstract

Rao, A.V., S. Agarwal. "Role of antioxidant lycopene in cancer and heart disease." *Journal of the American College of Nutrition,* October 2000; 19(5):563–569.
http://www.ncbi.nlm.nih.gov/entrez/query.fcgi?cmd=Retrieve&db=PubMed&list=_uid s=11022869&dopt=Abstract

Ravnskov, U. "Diet-heart disease hypothesis is wishful thinking." *British Medical Journal,* January 26, 2002; 324:238.
http://www.ncbi.nlm.nih.gov/entrez/query.fcgi?cmd=Retrieve&db=PubMed&list=_uid s=11809658&dopt=Abstract

Reda, T.K., A. Geliebter, F.X. Pi-Sunyer. "Amylin, food intake, and obesity." *Obesity Research,* October 2002; 10(10): 1087–1091.
http://www.ncbi.nlm.nih.gov/entrez/query.fcgi?cmd=Retrieve&db=PubMed&list=_uids =12376591&dopt=Abstract

Ridker, P.M., C.H. Hennekens, J.E. Buring, N. Rifai. "C-reactive protein and other markers of inflammation in the prediction of cardiovascular disease in women." *New England Journal of Medicine,* March 23, 2000; 342:836–843.
http://www.ncbi.nlm.nih.gov/entrez/query.fcgi?cmd=Retrieve&db=PubMed&list=_uid s=10733371&dopt=Abstract

Roberts, S.B. "High-glycemic index foods, hunger, and obesity: is there a connection?" *Nutrition Reviews,* June 2000; 58(6):163–169.
http://www.ncbi.nlm.nih.gov/entrez/query.fcgi?cmd=Retrieve&db=PubMed&list=_uid s=10885323&dopt=Abstract

Schwarz, J.M., P. Linfoot, D. Dare, K. Aghajanian. "Hepatic de novo lipogenesis in normoinsulinemic and hyperinsulinemic subjects consuming high-fat, low-carbohydrate and low-fat, high-carbohydrate isoenergetic diets." *American Journal of Clinical Nutrition,* January 2003; 77(1):43–50.
http://www.ncbi.nlm.nih.gov/entrez/query.fcgi?cmd=Retrieve&db=PubMed&list=_uid s=12499321&dopt=Abstract

Simoneau, J.A., J.H. Veerkamp, L.P. Turcotte, D.E. Kelley. "Markers of capacity to utilize fatty acids in human skeletal muscle: relation to insulin resistance and effects of weight loss." *FASEB Journal* 1999; 13:2051–2060.
http://www.ncbi.nlm.nih.gov/entrez/query.fcgi?cmd=Retrieve&db=PubMed&list=_uids=10544188&dopt=Abstract

Stoll, B.A. "Upper abdominal obesity, insulin resistance and breast cancer risk." *International Journal of Obesity Related Metabolic Disorder,* June 2002; 26(6): 747–753.
http://www.ncbi.nlm.nih.gov/entrez/query.fcgi?cmd=Retrieve&db=PubMed&list=_uids=12037643&dopt=Abstract

Torre, P., S. Fusco, F. Quaglia, et al. "Immune response of the coeliac nasal mucosa to locally-instilled gliadin." *Clinical Experimental Immunology*, March 2002; 127(3):513–518.
http://www.ncbi.nlm.nih.gov/entrez/query.fcgi?cmd=Retrieve&db=PubMed&list=_uids=11966769&dopt=Abstract

Tucker, K.L., H. Chen, M.T. Hannan, et al. "Bone mineral density and dietary patterns in older adults: the Framingham Osteoporosis Study." *American Journal of Clinical Nutrition,* July 2002; 76(1):245–252.
http://www.ncbi.nlm.nih.gov/entrez/query.fcgi?cmd=Retrieve&db=PubMed&list=_uids=12081842&dopt=Abstract

Valentino, R., S. Savastano, M. Maglio, et al. "Markers of potential coeliac disease in patients with Hashimoto's thyroiditis." *European Journal of Endocrinology,* April 2002; 146(4):479–483.
http://www.ncbi.nlm.nih.gov/entrez/query.fcgi?cmd=Retrieve&db=PubMed&list=_uids=11916614&dopt=Abstract

Willett, W., J. Manson, S. Liu. "Glycemic index, glycemic load, and risk of type 2 diabetes." *American Journal of Clinical Nutrition,* July 2002; 76(1):274S–280S.
http://www.ncbi.nlm.nih.gov/entrez/query.fcgi?cmd=Retrieve&db=PubMed&list=_uids=12081851&dopt=Abstract

Chapter Three

Bray, G.A., J.C. Lovejoy, S.R. Smith, et al. "The influence of different fats and fatty acids on obesity, insulin resistance and inflammation." *Journal of Nutrition,* September 2002; 132(9):2488–2491.
http://www.ncbi.nlm.nih.gov/entrez/query.fcgi?cmd=Retrieve&db=PubMed&list=_uids=12221198&dopt=Abstract

Colhoun, H.M. "The big picture on obesity and insulin resistance." *Journal of the American College of Cardiology,* September 4, 2002; 40(5):944–945.
http://www.ncbi.nlm.nih.gov/entrez/query.fcgi?cmd=Retrieve&db=PubMed&list=_uids =12225720&dopt=Abstract

Cummings, D.E., M.W. Schwartz. "Genetics and Pathophysiology of Human Obesity." *Annual Review of Medicine,* October 28, 2002.
http://www.ncbi.nlm.nih.gov/entrez/query.fcgi?cmd=Retrieve&db=PubMed&list=_uids =12414915&dopt=Abstract

Elliott, S.S., N.L. Keim, J.S. Stern, et al. "Fructose, weight gain, and the insulin resistance syndrome." *American Journal of Clinical Nutrition,* November 2002; 76(5):911–922.
http://www.ncbi.nlm.nih.gov/entrez/query.fcgi?cmd=Retrieve&db=PubMed&list=_uids =12399260&dopt=Abstract

Ivandic, A., I. Prpic-Krizevac, D. Bozic, et al. "Insulin resistance and androgens in healthy women with different body fat distributions." *Wien Klin Wochenschr,* May 15, 2002; 114(8–9):321–326.
http://www.ncbi.nlm.nih.gov/entrez/query.fcgi?cmd=Retrieve&db=PubMed&list=_uids =12212367&dopt=Abstract

O'Rahilly, S. "Insights into obesity and insulin resistance from the study of extreme human phenotypes." *European Journal Endocrinology,* October 2002; 147(4):435–441.
http://www.ncbi.nlm.nih.gov/entrez/query.fcgi?cmd=Retrieve&db=PubMed&list=_uids =12370103&dopt=Abstract

Porte, D., Jr., D.G. Baskin, M.W. Schwartz. "Leptin and insulin action in the central nervous system." *Nutrition Review,* October 2002; 60(10 Pt 2):S20–29; discussion S68–84, 85–87.
http://www.ncbi.nlm.nih.gov/entrez/query.fcgi?cmd=Retrieve&db=PubMed&list=_uids =12403080&dopt=Abstract

Scarpace, P.J., M. Matheny, Y. Zhang, et al. "Leptin-Induced Leptin Resistance Reveals Separate Roles for the Anorexic and Thermogenic Responses in Weight Maintenance." *Endocrinology,* August 2002, Vol. 143, No. 8, 3026–3035.
http://endo.endojournals.org/cgi/content/abstract/143/8/3026

USDA Food Pyramid Guide
http://www.pueblo.gsa.gov/cic=_text/food/food-pyramid/main.htm

Chapter Four

Oschman, James L. and Churchill Livingstone. *Energy Medicine*. Harcourt Publishers Limited, 2000.

Chapter Five

Hoogwerf, B.J., D.L. Sprecher, G.L Pearce. "Blood glucose concentrations < or = 125 mg/dl and coronary heart disease risk." *American Journal of Cardiology*, March 2002(1); 89(5):596–599.
http://www.ncbi.nlm.nih.gov/entrez/query.fcgi?cmd=Retrieve&db=PubMed&list=_uids =11867048&dopt=Abstract

O'Reilly, D.J. "Thyroid function tests—time for a reassessment." *British Medical Journal*, May 13, 2000; 320:1332–1334.
http://bmj.com/cgi/content/full/320/7245/1332

Zhu, S., Z. Wang, S. Heshka, et al. "Waist circumference and obesity-associated risk factors among whites in the third National Health and Nutrition Examination Survey: clinical action thresholds." *American Journal of Clinical Nutrition*, October 2002; 76:743–749.
http://www.ncbi.nlm.nih.gov/entrez/query.fcgi?cmd=Retrieve&db=PubMed&list=_uids =12324286&dopt=Abstract

Chapter Seven

Andersen, J.H., M.E. Poulsen. "Results from the monitoring of pesticide residues in fruit and vegetables on the Danish market, 1998–99." *Food Additives and Contaminants*, October 2001; 18(10):906–931.
http://www.ncbi.nlm.nih.gov/entrez/query.fcgi?cmd=Retrieve&db=PubMed&list=_uids =11569771&dopt=Abstract

Aronson, W.J., J.A. Glaspy, S.T. Reddy, et al. "Modulation of omega-3/omega-6 polyunsaturated ratios with dietary fish oils in men with prostate cancer." *Urology*, August 2001; 58(2):283–288.
http://www.ncbi.nlm.nih.gov/entrez/query.fcgi?cmd=Retrieve&db=PubMed&list=_uids =11489728&dopt=Abstract

Baker, B.P., C.M. Benbrook, E. Groth, et al. "Pesticide residues in conventional, IPM-grown and organic foods: Insights from three U.S. data sets." *Food Additives and Contaminants*, May 2002; 19(5):427–446.

http://www.ncbi.nlm.nih.gov/entrez/query.fcgi?cmd=Retrieve&db=PubMed&list=_uids =12028642&dopt=Abstract

Bolger, P.M., B.A. Schwetz. "Mercury and health." *New England Journal of Medicine,* November 28, 2002; 347(22):1735–1736.
http://www.ncbi.nlm.nih.gov/entrez/query.fcgi?cmd=Retrieve&db=PubMed&list=_uids =12456847&dopt=Abstract

Carrington, C.D., M.P. Bolger. "An exposure assessment for methylmercury from seafood for consumers in the United States." *Risk Analysis,* August 2002; 22(4):689–699.
http://www.ncbi.nlm.nih.gov/entrez/query.fcgi?cmd=Retrieve&db=PubMed&list=_uids =12224743&dopt=Abstract

Holub, B. "Omega-3 fatty acids in cardiovascular care." *Canadian Medical Association Journal,* March 5, 2002; 166:608–615.
http://www.cmaj.ca/cgi/content/full/166/5/608?maxtoshow=&HITS=10&hits=10&R ESULTFORMAT=&searchid=1037565774474_2452&stored_search=&FIRSTINDEX =0&volume=166&firstpage=608&journalcode=cmaj

Hightower, J.M. "Mercury Levels in High-End Consumers of Fish." *Environmental Health Perspectives,* November 1, 2002.
http://ehpnet1.niehs.nih.gov/docs/2003/5837/abstract.html

Kim, Y., S.K. Ji, H. Choi. "Modulation of liver microsomal monooxygenase system by dietary n-6/n-3 ratios in rat hepatocarcinogenesis." *Nutrition Cancer,* 2000; 37(1):65–72.
http://www.ncbi.nlm.nth.gov/entrez/query.fcgi?cmd=Retrieve&db=PubMed&list=_uids =10965521&dopt=Abstract

Liu, G., D.M. Bibus, A.M. Bode, et al. "Omega 3 but not omega 6 fatty acids inhibit AP-1 activity and cell transformation in JB6 cells." *Proceedings National Academy Science USA,* June 19, 2001; 98(13):7510–7515.
http://www.pubmedcentral.gov/articlerender.fcgi?tool=pubmed&pubmedid=11416221

Maillard, V., P. Bougnoux, P. Ferrari, et al. "N-3 and N-6 fatty acids in breast adipose tissue and relative risk of breast cancer in a case-control study in Tours, France." *International Journal of Cancer,* March 2002; 98(1):78–83.
http://www.ncbi.nlm.nih.gov/entrez/query.fcgi?cmd=Retrieve&db=PubMed&list=_uids =11857389&dopt=Abstract

Mercola, J.M. "Omega-3's and Childhood Asthma." *Thorax,* March 2002; 57 (3)281.
http://www.ncbi.nlm.nih.gov/entrez/query.fcgi?cmd=Retrieve&db=PubMed&list=_uids =11867839&dopt=Abstract

Peterson, S.A., A.T. Herlihy, R.M. Hughes, et al. "Level and extent of mercury contamination in Oregon, USA, lotic fish." *Environmental Toxicology Chemical*, October 2002; 21(10):2157–2164.
http://www.ncbi.nlm.nih.gov/entrez/query.fcgi?cmd=Retrieve&db=PubMed&list=_uids =12371492&dopt=Abstract

Slattery, M.L., J. Benson, K.N. Ma, et al. "Trans-fatty acids and colon cancer." *Nutrition Cancer,* 2001; 39(2):170–5.
http://www.ncbi.nlm.nih.gov/entrez/query.fcgi?cmd=Retrieve&db=PubMed&list=_uids =11759276&dopt=Abstract

Wooltorton, E. "Facts on mercury and fish consumption." *Canadian Medical Association Journal*, October 15, 2002; 167(8):897.
http://www.cmaj.ca/cgi/content/full/167/8/897?maxtoshow=&HITS=10&hits=10&R ESULTFORMAT=&searchid=1037374696248_1118&stored_search=&FIRSTINDEX =0&volume=167&firstpage=897&journalcode=cmaj

Chapter Nine

Blanchard, G., B.M. Paragon, F. Milliat, et al. "Dietary L-carnitine supplementation in obese cats alters carnitine metabolism and decreases ketosis during fasting and induced hepatic lipidosis." *Journal of Nutrition*, February 2002; 132(2):204–210.
http://www.ncbi.nlm.nih.gov/entrez/query.fcgi?cmd=Retrieve&db=PubMed&list=_uid s=11823579&dopt=Abstract

Bretherton-Watt, D., R. Given-Wilson, J.L. Mansi, et al. "Vitamin D receptor gene polymorphisms are associated with breast cancer risk in a UK Caucasian population." *British Journal of Cancer*, July 2001 20; 85(2):171–175.
http://www.ncbi.nlm.nih.gov/entrez/query.fcgi?cmd=Retrieve&db=PubMed&list=_uid s=11461072&dopt=Abstract

Chan, J., S.F. Knutsen, G.G. Blix, et al. "Water, other fluids, and fatal coronary heart disease: the Adventist Health Study." *American Journal of Epidemiology*, May 2002; 155(9):827–833.
http://www.ncbi.nlm.nih.gov/entrez/query.fcgi?cmd=Retrieve&db=PubMed&list=_uid s=11978586&dopt=Abstract

Erren, T.C., C. Piekarski. "Light and life—facts and research perspectives at the Cologne Light Symposium 2002." *Neuroendocrinology Letters,* July 2002; 23 Suppl 2:4–6.
http://www.ncbi.nlm.nih.gov/entrez/query.fcgi?cmd=Retrieve&db=PubMed&list=_uid s=12163840&dopt=Abstract

Francois, C.A., S.L. Connor, L.C. Bolewicz, W.E. Connor. "Supplementing lactating women with flaxseed oil does not increase docosahexaenoic acid in their milk." *American Journal of Clinical Nutrition,* January 2003; 77: 226–233.
http://www.ncbi.nlm.nih.gov/entrez/query.fcgi?cmd=Retrieve&db=PubMed&list=_uid s=12499346&dopt=Abstract

French, P.W., R. Penny, J.A. Laurence, et al. "Mobile phones, heat shock proteins and cancer." *Differentiation,* June 2001; 67(4–5):93–97.
http://www.ncbi.nlm.nih.gov/entrez/query.fcgi?cmd=Retrieve&db=PubMed&list=_uid s=11683499&dopt=Abstract

Gandhi, O.P. "Electromagnetic fields: human safety issues." *Annual Review Biomedical Engineering,* 2002; 4:211–234.
http://www.ncbi.nlm.nih.gov/entrez/query.fcgi?cmd=Retrieve&db=PubMed&list=_uids =12117757&dopt=Abstract

Garssen, J., H. van Loveren. "Effects of ultraviolet exposure on the immune system." *Critical Reviews Immunology,* 2001; 21(4):359–397.
http://www.ncbi.nlm.nih.gov/entrez/query.fcgi?cmd=Retrieve&db=PubMed&list=_uids =11922079&dopt=Abstract

Gonzalez-Ortiz, M., E. Martinez-Abundis, et al. "Effect of sleep deprivation on insulin sensitivity and cortisol concentration in healthy subjects." *Diabetes Nutrition Metabolism,* April 2000; 13(2):80–83.
http://www.ncbi.nlm.nih.gov/entrez/query.fcgi?cmd=Retrieve&db=PubMed&list=_uids =10898125&dopt=Abstract

Grover, J.K., S. Yadav, V. Vats. "Medicinal plants of India with anti-diabetic potential." *Journal of Ethnopharmacology,* June 2002; 81(1):81–100.
http://www.ncbi.nlm.nih.gov/entrez/query.fcgi?cmd=Retrieve&db=PubMed&list=_uids =12020931&dopt=Abstract

Harada, S., Y. Kasahara. "Inhibitory effect of gurmarin on palatal taste responses to amino acids in the rat." *American Journal of Physiology. Regulatory, Integrative and Comparative Physiology,* June 2000; 278(6):R1513–1517.

Heaney, R.P., K.M. Davies, T.C. Chen, et al. "Human serum 25-hydroxycholecalciferol response to extended oral dosing with cholecalciferol." *American Journal of Clinical Nutrition,* January 2003; 77(1):204–210.
http://www.ncbi.nlm.nih.gov/entrez/query.fcgi?cmd=Retrieve&db=PubMed&list=_uids =12499343&dopt=Abstract

Hirsch, J. "The search for new ways to treat obesity." *Proceedings National Academy Science USA,* July 9, 2002; 99(14):9096–9097.
http://www.ncbi.nlm.nih.gov/entrez/query.fcgi?cmd=Retrieve&db=PubMed&list=_uids =12093927&dopt=Abstract

Iimuro, M., H. Shibata, T. Kawamori, et al. "Suppressive effects of garlic extract on Helicobacter pylori-induced gastritis in Mongolian gerbils." *Cancer Letters*, December 10, 2002; 187(1–2):61.
http://www.ncbi.nlm.nih.gov/entrez/query.fcgi?cmd=Retrieve&db=PubMed&list=_uids =12359352&dopt=Abstract

Jakicic, J.M., R.R. Wing, C. Winters-Hart. "Relationship of physical activity to eating behaviors and weight loss in women." *Medicine & Science in Sports & Exercise,* October 2002; 34(10):1653–1659.
http://www.ncbi.nlm.nih.gov/entrez/query.fcgi?cmd=Retrieve&db=PubMed&list=_uids =12370568&dopt=Abstract

Kreiter, S.R., R.P. Schwartz, H.N. Kirkman, Jr., et al. "Nutritional rickets in African American breast-fed infants." *Journal of Pediatrics*, August 2000; 137(2):153–157.
http://www.ncbi.nlm.nih.gov/entrez/query.fcgi?cmd=Retrieve&db=PubMed&list=_uids =10931404&dopt=Abstract

Lambert, G.W., C. Reid, D.M. Kaye, et al. "Effect of sunlight and season on serotonin turnover in the brain." *Lancet,* December 7, 2002; 360(9348):1840–1842.
http://www.thelancet.com/journal/vol360/iss9348/full/llan.360.9348.original_ research.23462.1

Makishima, M., T.T. Lu, W. Xie, et al. "Vitamin D receptor as an intestinal bile acid sensor." *Science*, May 17, 2002; 296(5571):1313–1316.
http://www.ncbi.nlm.nih.gov/entrez/query.fcgi?cmd=Retrieve&db=PubMed&list=_uids =12016314&dopt=Abstract

Murphy, M., A. Nevill, C. Neville. "Accumulating brisk walking for fitness, cardiovascular risk, and psychological health." *Medicine & Science in Sports & Exercise*, September 2002; 34:1468–1474.
http://www.ncbi.nlm.nih.gov/entrez/query.fcgi?cmd=Retrieve&db=PubMed&list=_uids =12218740&dopt=Abstract

Parry, B.L. "Jet lag: minimizing its effects with critically timed bright light and melatonin administration." *Journal of Molecular Microbiology and Biotechnology*, September 2002; 4(5):463–646.
http://www.ncbi.nlm.nih.gov/entrez/query.fcgi?cmd=Retrieve&db=PubMed&list=_uids =12432956&dopt=Abstract

Perkowitz, S. "The physics of light and sunlight." *Neuroendocrinology Letters*, July 2002; 23 Suppl 2:14–16.
http://www.ncbi.nlm.nih.gov/entrez/query.fcgi?cmd=Retrieve&db=PubMed&list=_uids =12163842&dopt=Abstract

Renaud, S., D. Lanzmann-Petithory. "Dietary fats and coronary heart disease pathogenesis." *Current Atheroscler Report,* November 2002; 4(6):419–424.
http://www.ncbi.nlm.nih.gov/entrez/query.fcgi?cmd=Retrieve&db=PubMed&list=_uid s=12361488&dopt=Abstract

Riserus, U., L. Berglund, B. Vessby. "Conjugated linoleic acid (CLA) reduced abdominal adipose tissue in obese middle-aged men with signs of the metabolic syndrome: a randomised controlled trial." *International Journal of Obesity Related Metabolic Disorders,* August 2001; 25(8):1129–1135.
http://www.ncbi.nlm.nih.gov/entrez/query.fcgi?cmd=Retrieve&db=PubMed&list=_uid s=11477497&dopt=Abstract

Roberts, C.K., N.D. Vaziri, R.J. Barnard. "Effect of diet and exercise intervention on blood pressure, insulin, oxidative stress, and nitric oxide availability." *Circulation,* November 12, 2002; 106(20):2530–2532.
http://www.ncbi.nlm.nih.gov/entrez/query.fcgi?cmd=Retrieve&db=PubMed&list=_uid s=12427646&dopt=Abstract

Rogers, N.L., M.P. Szuba, J.P. Staab, et al. "Neuroimmunologic aspects of sleep and sleep loss." *Seminars Clinical Neuropsychiatry,* October 2001; 6(4):295–307.
http://www.ncbi.nlm.nih.gov/entrez/query.fcgi?cmd=Retrieve&db=PubMed&list=_uid s=11607924&dopt=Abstract

Ross, R., D. Dagnone, P.J. Jones, et al. "Reduction in Obesity and Related Comorbid Conditions after Diet-Induced Weight Loss or Exercise-Induced Weight Loss in Men. A Randomized, Controlled Trial." *Annals of Internal Medicine,* July 2000; 133:92–103.
http://www.annals.org/issues/v133n2/full/200007180-00008.html

Rothman, K.J. "Epidemiological evidence on health risks of cellular telephones." *Lancet,* November 25, 2000; 356(9244):1837–1840.
http://www.ncbi.nlm.nih.gov/entrez/query.fcgi?cmd=Retrieve&db=PubMed&list=_uid s=11117928&dopt=Abstract

Sheehy, C.M., P.A. Perry, S.L. Cromwell. "Dehydration: biological considerations, age-related changes, and risk factors in older adults." *Biological Research Nursing,* July 1999; 1(1):30–37.
http://www.ncbi.nlm.nih.gov/entrez/query.fcgi?cmd=Retrieve&db=PubMed&list=_uid s=11225294&dopt=Abstract

Smith, J.S., D.F. Kripke, J.A. Elliott, et al. "Illumination of upper and middle visual fields produces equivalent suppression of melatonin in older volunteers." *Chronobiology International,* September 2002; 19(5):883–891.
http://www.ncbi.nlm.nih.gov/entrez/query.fcgi?cmd=Retrieve&db=PubMed&list=_uid s=12405551&dopt=Abstract

Spiegel, K., R. Leproult, E. Van Cauter. "Impact of sleep debt on metabolic and endocrine function." *Lancet,* October 23, 1999; 354:1435–1439.
http://www.ncbi.nlm.nih.gov/entrez/query.fcgi?cmd=Retrieve&db=PubMed&list=_uid s=10543671&dopt=Abstract

Tangpricha, V., E.N. Pearce, T.C. Chen, M.F. Holick. "Vitamin D insufficiency among free-living healthy young adults." *American Journal of Medicine,* June 1, 2002; 112(8):659–662.
http://www.ncbi.nlm.nih.gov/entrez/query.fcgi?cmd=Retrieve&db=PubMed&list=_uid s=12034416&dopt=Abstract

Vgontzas, A.N., E.O. Bixler, H.M. Lin, et al. "Chronic insomnia is associated with nyctohemeral activation of the hypothalamic-pituitary-adrenal axis: clinical implications." *Journal Clinical Endocrinology Metabolism,* August 2001; 86(8):3787–3794.
http://www.ncbi.nlm.nih.gov/entrez/query.fcgi?cmd=Retrieve&db=PubMed&list=_uid s=11502812&dopt=Abstract

Chapters Ten and Eleven

www.emofree.com and conversations with Gary Craig, EFT founder.

Chapters Eight and Twelve

Most of the recipes and menu plans were initially devised by nutritionist Gabrielle Rabner and Alison Rose Levy in close consultation with Dr. Mercola. Chef Nancy Davin created additional recipes and recipe variations. She also taste-tested all of the recipes, and finalized the flavors and all recipe ingredients and instructions.

NO-GRAIN RESOURCES

Recommended Websites

www.nograindiet.com

As you go *No-Grain,* you'll find that there's a whole world of resources there for you, and one of the most exciting is my free website, *www.nograindiet.com,* designed to be interactive with this book. My aim is to leverage the incredible power of the Internet, to continue to bring you the most current resources and tools so you can successfully implement—and maintain—all the strategies in this book.

www.nograindiet.com contains thousands of pages of useful health information, the latest information relevant to the *No-Grain* lifestyle, creating a community of participants and experts you can call on at any time. So don't forget to check the site regularly for recipes, exercises, EFT strategies, as well as continually updated contacts for EFT practitioners, with ratings provided by former clients. I encourage you to check out *www.nograindiet.com* once you complete this book, as this is sure to become an important resource in your health program.

www.westonaprice.org

This site is dedicated to the research of nutrition pioneer Dr. Weston Price, whose studies of isolated nonindustrialized peoples have helped physicians home in on optimal human diets. Dr. Price's research demonstrated that humans achieve perfect physical form and perfect health generation after generation only when they consume nutrient-dense whole foods and the vital fat-soluble activators found exclusively in animal fats.

www.price-pottenger.org

This site is also provides information on Dr. Price, as well as Dr. Francis Pottenger, another pioneering nutritional researcher.

Recommended Books

Most of my recommendations are available at your library. However, you can also find more extensive reviews, as well as links to purchase, at *www.nograindiet.com*.

Metabolic Typing Diet
William Wolcott

All of the patients in my clinic are metabolically typed, which helps me to individualize their diet programs. Author William Wolcott spent over twenty-five years developing this program, which is incredibly helpful for those who fail to respond to more general recommendations.

Dangerous Grains
James Braly, M.D.

A recently published book that will open your eyes to the impact of gluten grains on chronic illness such as cancer, autoimmune disease, osteoporosis, and intestinal diseases. Gluten sensitivity affects tens of millions of Americans and is easily corrected by grain restriction or elimination.

The Recipe For Living Without Disease
Aajonus Vanderplanitz

For most of us, raw foods are key to optimizing health. Aajonus is the only raw food animal proponent I know of, and his recent book is a wonderful resource of wisdom on how to include more of the ultimate fast food in our diet—uncooked foods.

Nutrition and Physical Degeneration
Weston Price, D.D.S.

One of the major nutritional pioneers of the twentieth century, Dr. Price traveled around the globe documenting the effects of diet on health and disease. The pictures alone are worth the price of the book. A must for every serious student of nutrition and health.

The Omega-3 Connection
Andrew Stoll, M.D.

Dr. Stoll is the director of the psychopharmacology research lab at Boston's McLean Hospital and assistant professor of psychiatry at Harvard Medical School. He discusses the use of omega-3 extensively in his book and reviews the new evidence supporting the use of omega-3 oils for mental illness and other chronic degenerative diseases.

The Paleo Diet
Loren Cordain, Ph.D.

Dr. Cordain is considered one of the world's leading experts on Paleolithic (Stone Age) nutrition. He has compiled an easy to understand, authoritative reference on the scientific documentation for reducing our grain consumption to be more in line with our ancient ancestors.

Life Without Bread
Wolfgang Lutz, M.D.

Dr. Lutz is a physician who has had great success with thousands of patients in his private practice in Germany. He has compiled an amazing amount of comprehensive long-term information on low-carbohydrate nutrition's impact on health and disease.

Trust Us, We're Experts: How Industry Manipulates Science and Gambles with Your Future
Sheldon Rampton and John Stauber

If you have any interest in understanding how our society has been inundated with misinformation on how grains affect health—and a variety of other issues that the media attempts to deceive us on—then I highly recommend this book.

EFT Resources

www.nograindiet.com

You can obtain a free extended report with full pictures on how to actually perform EFT by going to *www.nograindiet.com*. There is also an extended section on using EFT specifically for weight loss and other positive goals in your life, such as increasing your exercise, improved relationships, and increased income or material possessions.

There are also videos on EFT that can be purchased for more comprehensive instruction.

We hope to have an extensive list of EFT practitioners on the site that have been rated by others who have seen them so you will have an easy way to see what others are saying about the therapists. In many ways it will be similar to the reviews on *amazon.com*.

www.emofree.com

This is Gary Craig's website. He is the developer of EFT and has many thousands of pages that document the widespread use of EFT. The many examples also serve as powerful teaching examples. His free newsletter is an absolute must if you have any interest in EFT.

Gary also has an extensive list of practitioners on his site. However, none of them have been certified or have any evaluations. If the practitioner rating section of *www.nograindiet.com* is not available by the time this book is published, you can use Gary's list as a convenient starting point for finding an EFT therapist.

www.eftupdate.com

Dr. Patricia Carrington has also compiled a very helpful set of EFT resources on her site. She has worked closely with Gary Craig over the years and has created an enhancement of EFT called Choices that provides additional options that can be used with EFT.

She also has a list of practitioners that have passed an EFT Certificate of Completion (EFT-CC) Examination—evidence that they have studied and fully understand Gary Craig's Basic EFT Home Study Course (thirteen videos on CD, one audio on CD, and one instruction manual). The list does not, however, give you any information about the competence with which the practitioner applies EFT.

www.eftsupport.com

This is another site run by Dr. Patricia Carrington that is designed to provide support for those people who know EFT. She also has a regular newsletter with many terrific real-world examples.

www.energypsych.org

The Association for Comprehensive Energy Psychology (ACEP) is the professional organization that coordinates energy psychology. If you are a health care professional wishing to learn more about other energy psychology techniques or professional annual spring conferences, you will be able to learn about future conferences here.

www.meridianpsych.com

Dr. Sharon Cass Toole coordinates the other energy psychology conference, typically held in Toronto in November. Details of future conferences are posted on her site.

Nutritional Resources

Metabolic Typing

Virtually all of my patients are implementing the Metabolic Typing program as developed by William Wolcott at Healthexcel. If you are not achieving the results you would like with the *No-Grain Diet,* there is a possibility that you are a very slow oxidizer or strongly "sympathetically dominant." If this is the case I would encourage you to obtain a copy of the *Metabolic Typing Diet* book and perform the basic test in the book, as it will provide you with a way to confirm this. You will then be able to customize your *No-Grain Diet* program to your unique needs.

In my office I do the Intermediate Metabolic Typing Program testing via an on-line questionnaire that is analyzed by a sophisticated computer program. The analysis is then transmitted as a twenty-five-page report that details one's metabolic type and requirements.

I have three nutritionists in my office who then review the results of the Metabolic Typing Test with my patients. This allows us to individualize their diet so it is optimized for their individual biochemistry.

For our more seriously ill patients, we perform the Advanced Metabolic Type Program that involves a variety of biochemical challenges and physical monitoring tools, such as body temperature readings, blood sugar responses to oral glucose challenges, along with urine and saliva pH testing.

I am in the process of facilitating a training program so trained clinicians are available to serve as Metabolic Typing consultants. I hope to have this available by the late spring or summer of 2003.

You can go to either *www.mercola.com* or *www.nograindiet.com* to learn the current status of the Metabolic Typing program. If the program is not yet in place, you can sign up for the newsletter on either site and you will receive a notification as to when that will be available.

INDEX

ACKNOWLEDGMENTS

"If I have seen further it is by standing on the shoulders of giants."
—Sir Isaac Newton 1676

Seeking the truth and applying it to life to improve health has been a passion of mine since I was in grade school. It is quite clear that Sir Isaac Newton had it right when he observed that teachers are essential for us to make any significant progress.

My first mentor was my loving mother, whose nonjudgmental, uncritical, and constant love provided a solid foundation that helped me develop many of the strategies that you will read about in this book. Most important, she helped to nurture my relationship with my Creator. I consider that the most significant and influential factor that has structured my life. God's grace has been outrageously abundant in my life and is instrumental in helping me bring these concepts to you.

My first health instructor was Dr. Kenneth Cooper. I first read his book *Aerobics* in 1968 and have been exercising regularly ever since then. He helped me understand the importance that regular body movement has in optimizing health.

Dr. William Crook, who wrote the popular book *The Yeast Connection,* provided me with the first clue that grains might actually contribute to disease in some people. He passed away at eighty-five years of age, as the manuscript for this book was being completed, and he will be missed. His book also provided a connection to Dr. Gary Oberg, former president of the American Academy of Environmental Medicine, who was kind enough to spend some time with me early in my career and helped me network with other nutritionally minded physicians.

One of these physicians was Dr. Tom Stone, an early electrodermal and nutritional pioneer in the Chicago area. He was a major influence in my transition out of the traditional medical paradigm.

In 1995 Dr. Ron Rosedale expanded my understanding of the negative influence of grains and insulin on health and on weight management.

Dr. Dietrich Klinghardt was also an early mentor and guide, providing a deeper understanding of health and disease; his friendship is sincerely appreciated. He also indirectly led to the development of this book by providing the connection with the book's coauthor, Alison Rose Levy.

Alison is the primary reason *The No-Grain Diet* was written. Her initiative and skill in transforming clinical truths into clear and motivating content is the main reason it is so practical and helpful. She also helped connect me with my literary agent, Janis Vallely, whose expertise and highly professional approach are major reasons the book now exists. Deep appreciation is also extended to Brian Tart at Dutton, whose wisdom and guidance have been essential in crafting this book.

To date, the most valuable healing gift I have been given in medicine is a form of psychological acupressure called Emotional Freedom Technique, and I am enormously grateful to Gary Craig, who developed EFT, for making this astonishing tool available to so many. We share similar visions and passions, and I am sincerely thankful for his friendship and kind assistance in helping with this book.

William Wolcott has developed Metabolic Typing over the past twenty-five years and has been very gracious in personally getting me up to speed with this valuable innovation in nutritional biochemistry.

Dr. Patricia Kane's assistance in ensuring the scientific accuracy of the text and in general editing is also greatly appreciated.

Just as important as my mentors are those who have helped me build the infrastructure to implement my vision. I have been in private practice since 1985 and have had the privilege of working with over one hundred wonderful employees. I wish to express my sincere appreciation for all their efforts in helping establish the Optimal Wellness Center.

I am especially appreciative of my sister Janet, who was my first office manager, for eleven years, until she retired to raise her children.

Meanwhile, my current office manager, Judy Kwasniewski, is a gift from God who somehow always ensures that everything runs smoothly. Our chief therapist, Jody Stevens, is a close and helpful friend whose support is appreciated both personally and professionally in our office, where she provides leadership in the emotional rebalancing that our wonderful staff of therapists perform.

My web team also does an awesome job of helping provide the best the Internet has to offer on health. Brian Vaszily, my chief web editor and an outstanding writer, has been instrumental in helping me position many of the points found on the site and in this book. Michael Valle's knowledge and insight have also been invaluable to the site's success. And my personal coach, Kirk Niemczyk, has helped me formulate the basic implementation strategies that led to the site and book in the first place.

Finally, I am most appreciative of the over twenty-thousand patients I have had the pleasure of serving as medical director of the Optimal Wellness Center. They truly are my greatest teachers, and I am enormously appreciative of their wisdom, patience, encouragement, and belief in me—they have been one of the greatest inspirations of all for this book, and for my life.

—*Dr. Joseph Mercola*

First of all, I want to thank Dr. Joseph Mercola for his positive energy, deep caring, and unbounded dedication to bringing Americans the best possible dietary and health wisdom. Brian Tart, our editor at Dutton, endowed this book with his clarity of focus from its inception. Janis Vallely, my/our literary agent, has been a true compass and a constant support in the ongoing creative process. Acknowledgment goes to Gabrielle Rabner for the many hours she devoted to the basic recipes and menu plans. I want to thank Chef Nancy Davin for refining, testing, and perfecting all the recipes, as well as contributing her mastery of international cuisine to our menu plans and the many delicious recipe variations.

I would also like to offer my gratitude to my grandmothers, whose love continues to smile down on me, from wherever they may be. Sadie encouraged my first, childhood attempts at cooking, and Anna clipped recipes and pasted them into my very first cookbook.

My late father, Henry Cohen, always encouraged me to believe that I had something of value to contribute to others, or as he put it, "to put my brick into the wall of the world." My mother, Evelyn Cohen, has instilled a sense of beauty and a passion for language, along with her unceasing love. My brother Dan tasted my first culinary efforts, and pointed out that ice cream should have sugar, not salt. His lifelong friendship and fraternity have been such a boon.

In the health arena, I have been incredibly fortunate to study with, and be mentored by, a few outstanding and pioneering doctors, teachers, and healers, to whom I owe my deepest gratitude. I bow my head in thanks to Bert Hellinger, Dr. Dietrich Klinghardt, Dr. Rudolph Ballentine, Dr. John Welwood, Harald Hohnen, Victoras Kulvinskas, Dr. Linda Bark, and John Friend, who continue to inspire and serve as the foundation for all my work.

To editors, catalysts, and colleagues who have generously provided direction and support in my professional path, I offer my warmest thanks: Jennifer Cook, Robert Owens Scott, Dena Vane, Kathryn Arnold, Matthew Solan, Peggy Bendet, Sheldon Lewis, Henry Dreher, Eden Marriott Kennedy, Melissa Scott, Jeannie Snyder, Marjorie Forman, and Sheila Saunders. Special thanks goes to Judith Asphar, and to Kitty Farmer, who introduced me both to my dear agent, Janis Vallely, and also to Dr. Dietrich Klinghardt, who has opened the doorways to healing.

I want to thank for their gift of loving friendship: William Eastman, Belleruth Naparstek, Bonnie and David Taylor, Bonnie Nelson Schwartz and the late Dr. David Abramson, Dan, Katherine, Anna and Rosalie Booth Cohen, Tom and Diane Durst, Patricia Davis, Lauren Versel Bresnan, and Zack Krieger and Linda Mapes.

Finally, I want to thank my husband, Ed, my team captain in the play of life and love.

—*Alison Rose Levy*

ABOUT THE AUTHORS

Dr. Joseph Mercola is an osteopathic physician; founder/director of *www.mercola.com*, one of the world's most visited health websites; and founder/director of The Optimal Wellness Center Medical Clinic just outside Chicago. Trained in both alternative and traditional medicine, he has served as the chairman of the family medicine department at St. Alexius Medical Center for five years. He lives in South Barrington, Illinois.

Alison Rose Levy is a freelance writer living in New York City.